The Clay Pedestal

The

Clay

Pedestal

A Re-examination of the

Doctor-Patient Relationship

Thomas Preston, M.D.

1981

MADRONA PUBLISHERS

SEATTLE

FIRST EDITION

10 9 8 7 6 5 4 3 2

Library of Congress Cataloging in Publication Data

Preston, Thomas A.
The clay pedestal.

Bibliography: p.
Includes index.
1. Physician and patient.   2. Medical errors.
I. Title.   [DNLM: 1. Physician-patient relations.
W 62 P941c]

R727.3.P73   610.69'6   81-11742
ISBN 0-914842-68-4   AACR2

Published by
Madrona Publishers, Inc.
2116 Western Avenue
Seattle, Washington 98121

We gratefully acknowledge permission to reprint the following material:
Richard Grossinger and Doubleday & Company, Inc. for material from *Planet
Medicine: The Art and Science of Healing Throughout the Ages* by Richard
Grossinger. Copyright © 1980 by Richard Grossinger. Reprinted by permission
of Doubleday & Company, Inc.

R 727
. 3
. P73

*To Micaela, Julie,
Cynthia, Terry, and Tom*

Author's Note

I URGE THE reader to note while reading this book, how frequently the most serious and consequential criticisms of modern medical practice come from physicians themselves, working and speaking through conventional medical forums. For the reader interested in more detailed analyses of the not-strictly-biological aspects of medicine, a bibliography is appended. Inevitably there are omissions, some of them of books which may have influenced me greatly. So extensive are writings in the medical field, by sociologists, economists, anthropologists, ethicists, and many others, that no doubt a totally different bibliography could substitute equally well for the one I have given.

I have tried to respect the English language, although in common with most physicians I find it often vexatious and demanding. And on one point I have submitted totally to tradition and the limitations of the language. There is no easy way to use the third person singular so as to refer to both sexes simultaneously, and I have chosen to follow the language rather than be intimidated by an awareness of its sexism.

I wish to thank Daniel Barr, Jill Severn, Malcolm Peterson and Linda Rosenstock, who persevered in reading early drafts and providing valuable direction. I thank especially Ann Adams, whose assistance made this book possible. And, lastly, I thank my publisher, who nurtured this project to reality.

THOMAS PRESTON

Seattle
July 1981

Contents

Introduction

EVEN AFTER twenty years in the medical profession, I marvel at the resourcefulness and intelligence of those who developed the knowledge and the technology that have given us a society in which good health is, for the most part, taken for granted. Just as impressive as the advances in science are the many doctors who apply this knowledge and technology to helping their patients. Their concern and compassion, and their devotion to the advancement of health and science frequently far exceeds my own capacity to give.

The notion of the consummate physician helping the distressed patient during his or her hour of need is undoubtedly the most enduring attraction for the public in its view of the medical profession. The power of that ideal was so strong for me that disillusionment with contemporary medical practices did not come easily. The myth of the selfless physician marshaling the forces of science for the welfare of his patients, however, has come to conceal reality rather than to reflect it, and to deflect inquiry into the true nature of medical practice, which falls far short of this mythical ideal.

Like many others given the privilege of practicing medicine, I perceive that we are not really doing our job as well as we should. Physicians enjoy privileges not given to members of most other occupations, and in return we are supposed to apply our skills and energies for the good of our patients. But in many respects we are not upholding that covenant.

It is difficult to get at the heart of what is wrong with medical care today, for those outside the profession don't understand the mechanisms and nuances of medical practice well enough to make an informed inquiry into it, and those within the profession seldom have the objectivity or detachment necessary to critically evaluate it. But behind the myth of medicine, the covenant between doctor and patient is, to an alarming extent, honored in the breach. The violation of the traditionally assumed contract between doctor and patient is only vaguely perceptible to a diffident public because of the mystification and obscurity of most medical practice.

The first time I saw a doctor talking a patient into an unnecessary operation, I believed the incident was an accident within a human system—the sort of accident that was bound to occur once in a while. A young surgeon, only months out of training, was desperate to operate, not only to produce income, but to exercise his skills and to "build up" his practice. The patient, a middle-aged man, had a weak knee, and the physical examination and X-rays showed no specific structural defect. The surgeon, with three of us medical students observing, told the patient, "If you want to keep walking on that knee you must have an operation." He gave the man no choice. Later he admitted to us under questioning that there was no guarantee the knee would be better, that it might be worse, but he was confident that he could strengthen the knee. The patient had the operation, which resulted in a stiffer and more painful knee. I knew already from observing my peers that some doctors saw medicine as an opportunity to gain wealth or prestige, but willful behavior for those ends was, I believed, very uncommon. So I saw the incident as isolated; an aberration as unintended but as inevitable as hemophilia or identical twinning.

Like most other medical students, I was slow to learn the ambiguity of clinical medicine, and I quite naturally attributed fatal outcomes to diseases incurable even by modern medicine. The first time I saw a patient die from what was clearly a physi-

cian's error—a collapsed lung inadvertently caused by unnecessarily trying to drain a small amount of fluid from around
the lung—I accepted the physician's defense of the act as "medically indicated," and the result as unpredictable and uncommon. I was consoled by the knowledge that even the best-trained
and most talented doctors are fallible. There is always some
uncertainty about the outcome of complex therapies and unpredictable diseases, and, for the most part, it seemed to me that
physicians gambled against death with Promethean courage.
Such losses, I understood, were personal and professional defeats for those responsible—defeats as unwelcome as a lost
battle is to an army general.

Because of the inevitability of death and the heroic triumphs I
saw around me, similar incidents were always easy enough to
see as the imperfections of men whose knowledge and skills I
still admired and hoped to emulate. Overwhelmed by the gravity
of the decisions we had to make, I regarded an occasional mistake or bad outcome as the lesser part of what was otherwise an
exhilarating and noble struggle against disease and death. In
medical school and during internships and residencies, my colleagues and I could not absorb that battlefield expertise fast
enough. Gradually, and with great effort, we became generals in
our own right. For us, as for those before us, the errors became
blurred by the rush of knowledge and the flush of partnership in
the great drama.

It was an experience fully seven years after graduation from
medical school that really made me question my thinking about
medicine. And even then, it was an experience that I would
come to understand only in retrospect.

I was standing in a group of physicians in a hospital corridor,
discussing a complex case that intrigued us as professionals and
dismayed us by its apparent insolubility. We listened with rapt
attention as the physician reporting the case began to speak with
great intensity. Just then, this physician was accosted by an
elderly patient who, with some trepidation, inquired about

when he would be able to go home from the hospital. The patient, a man in his late seventies who didn't exactly look as if he belonged to the ruling classes of America, managed in the same breath to explain that he had been trying for four hours to get information so that he could instruct his wife, who had to make arrangements with a friend to come and get him.

The interrupted physician turned on the old man in a rage, telling him to wait his turn during the doctor's rounds. "And besides," he shouted at the old man, "don't you see who you're interrupting?"

If any of us other physicians in that corridor felt indignation at the shameful behavior of our colleague, we didn't betray it, even in the expressions on our faces. For on this point, the code was clear: One physician does not interfere with another physician's professional relationships. But this time I could not excuse the behavior as a mistake or an aberration. The experience could not stand alone, for I had seen such arrogant and inhumane behavior too many times, in recurrent and diverse settings, and by physicians who, in private life, were friendly and well mannered.

Still, it was another ten years before I fully realized that what I had witnessed was not a personal trait, but a professional one. In the collective silence by which several physicians participated in the abuse of that elderly and weak man who sought only the fulfillment of our ancient vow to help him, we had expressed our devotion not to him, whom we claimed to serve, but to our own ideal: the notion of what we as physicians thought was best and what we wanted to do.

There is nothing congenitally wrong with the intelligent, industrious, and occasionally idealistic students who enter medical school that makes them turn out paternalistic at best, and, at worst, openly contemptuous of their patients. The explanation for physicians' arrogance is not in the individuals, but in the training they receive and in the structure of the professional setting. Somehow, in the process of becoming a physician, loyalty is focused on the profession that nurtures and sustains, and everything else becomes subordinated to that end—including the patient. Can there be any other explanation for the spectacle of doctors and their technologies keeping terminally ill patients alive and suffering far beyond the point of hope and the wishes of the anguished family? Is there another explanation for the physician's obsession with blood chemistry when what the patient needs is a little understanding and compassion? The medical subculture and its values are imposed on the physician, and he in turn imposes them on his patients.

The doctors' inability to sustain the ideal of devotion to their patients' interests, however, is only one component of the problem. There are others which, though less obvious, may be even more serious.

A second part of the malaise of contemporary medicine is the wholesale abuse and neglect of the scientific method. One need only to walk down a hospital hallway or attend a medical school lecture to hear the unscientific pronouncements, inaccurate conclusions, and delusions of infallibility all translated into medical practices that affect the lives and health of credulous patients. In medicine, the authority of physicians is so absolute that knowledge and the person who possesses it are one. Since the physician is regarded as a scientist, what he says is regarded as science itself, regardless of his methods or his proof. Professional solidarity prevents much questioning of such knowledge within the medical system.

Like most others learning medicine, I occasionally questioned a specific medical claim, but even when I was convinced of its incorrectness, I could always attribute the mistake to normal human error. But there is something repetitive about false claims in medicine, and eventually I saw the pattern, because I had practiced long enough to witness a full therapeutic cycle, which goes like this: A new therapy comes out, heralded at medical meetings and in the professional journals. Its creators become celebrities within the profession, and the media hail the advance. But after a period of euphoria and well-documented testimonials in support of the wonder treatment, a gradual disillusionment begins, lasting from a few months to a few decades. Then a new remedy is discovered, and, almost overnight, it replaces the old one, which is then summarily abandoned as worthless. What was once of certain benefit is now rejected. The cycle begins anew. It is not random human error that accounts for this phenomenon; on the contrary, it is a systematic deficiency of a medical system that substitutes the personal authority of physicians for scientific rigor.

Nor is it random chance that causes medical personnel and activity to be clustered in the practices that are most lucrative, without regard to patients' needs. That, too, is among the repetitive, systematic errors in medicine which must be understood if we are to change practices for the benefit of patients. These are inbred professional practices, and their magnitude and seriousness are scarcely imagined by the public.

To understand these errors we must understand their source: the profession, and the behavior of its member physicians. The power of physicians to intervene in the most crucial issues of life and death is far greater today than it was just fifty years ago, and so the need to understand and to change professional medical practices has become ever more urgent. Reform in medicine will be impossible without redefining and altering the status of the physician in our society and reshaping his role in medical decision-making.

Our inquiry into the nature of physicians must begin with the history of medicine, and particularly with the history of the relationship between sufferer and healer. The doctor-patient relationship is the crux of medical practice, and only through learning the nature and evolution of that relationship can patients improve their ability to get what they really need in encounters with physicians.

The doctor-patient relationship depends, in turn, on our beliefs about the role of therapy; that is, our beliefs about the curative powers of the healer. We must therefore study the elements that comprise the formula of healing, first as they were developed by the ancient physicians, and then as they have been used by quack doctors and healers of every stripe. We must see how these basic elements of healing have been incorporated into the modern physician's practice, and how they intermingle with conflicting scientific concepts. We must understand the physician's education and the process by which he is ordained into the profession, and how he gains by avoidance of public scrutiny of his acts.

We must understand the patient's role, and see how physicians and patients commonly work at cross-purposes because neither is fully aware of the interests and desires of the other.

We must examine what actually happens, not what we want to happen, in medical practice, if we are to understand the enormous waste of human resources and the danger to life and health that exists when the profession is not accountable to the public it serves.

And finally, the public must come to see its own hand in the formulation of medical practices, and its ability to produce change in the public interest. We must step back from the mystification of medicine to realize that much of it is political, social, and economic in nature, and that the public not only has a right to participate in medical decisions, but a responsibility to do so.

I acknowledge the undeniable relief of suffering brought to countless numbers of patients through the hard work, expertise and devotion of physicians everywhere. Also, I acknowledge the many honest physicians who are working hard to make medicine more scientific and humane. But their efforts are relatively small compared to the total of medical practice, and their pleas are largely ignored by most physicians. The critical remarks that follow are all the more difficult because of the basic goodwill of most physicians, and because of my own personal limitations in comparison to colleagues with whom I am in daily contact.

The Clay Pedestal

CHAPTER ONE

The Roots of Medical Practices

> These observances [physicians] impose because of the divine origin of disease, claiming superior knowledge and alleging other causes, so that, should the patient recover, the reputation for cleverness may be theirs; but should [he] die, they may have a sure fund of excuses, with the defence that they are not at all to blame, but the gods.
>
> Hippocrates

THE FUNDAMENTAL deception of medicine is the notion that doctors have special healing powers. This idea, held by doctors and patients alike, is embedded in our culture, with roots that go back to the beginning of medicine, and is the source of systematic errors in the practice of medicine.

Physicians today work in a setting unimagined by their predecessors of thousands of years ago—they discuss antibiotics, chromosomes, body scanners and other medical terms unknown just a hundred years ago—but the way they practice remains very much the same. It is popularly believed that to understand the workings of medicine, one must understand biology, genetics, human anatomy and physiology, and more recently, complex technology. But these are only a part of medicine, and the lesser part at that. The greater part is the way the doctor applies biological knowledge and technology to human illness. Open-heart surgery and drug treatment of cancer are of no value—indeed they are harmful—unless properly used. Medical practices are dictated by the attitudes of physicians. To understand these attitudes, we must look at the history of the profession, for the basic character of today's physician was formed deep in the past.

THE ANCIENT PHYSICIANS

Medicine in some form has very likely existed for as long as people have existed, if we accept as a definition of medicine care of the sick and wounded. Primitive native medicine, from which modern medicine evolved, is found in many parts of the world today, almost unchanged from its original form. Modern medicine has never totally replaced it even in Western countries, where the two have always been rivals.

Evidence of the practice of medicine dates back about thirty thousand years. A skull of that time has been found with a hole bored in it. That the operation (trephination) was not performed after death seems certain because there is new bone growth around the hole. Despite its striking resemblance to an operation performed by modern neurosurgeons, this trephination was probably done in order to release evil spirits the prehistoric surgeon believed were held captive, causing illness.

The oldest written medical records we have found are from ancient Egypt, beginning about 3500 B.C. The first doctor mentioned by name was Imhotep (circa 3000 B.C.), reputedly the builder of the first pyramids. The Egyptians were sophisticated enough to perform extensive surgery and practice internal medicine and ophthalmology. They acquired the habit, that is still with us, of using many drugs at the same time, presumably in the hope that if one didn't work, another might. The Babylonians devised tubes through which they could blow remedies into any human orifice. In fact, the most extensive system of medicine in antiquity flourished in Mesopotamia under the harsh laws of King Hammurabi, who wrote the first code of ethics for physicians. The ancient Assyrians provided free medical care for the poor, a forerunner of modern national health insurance.

Two important points emerge from our study of Egyptian and Mesopotamian medicine: (1) the practice of medicine was inseparable from religion, and (2) views about the nature and origin of diseases determined the actions of physicians. The ancients held the unambiguous belief that all illness resided in the hands of the gods, who were the sole restorers of health. As intermediary between the patient and the gods, the physician was essentially a priest. Thoth (known as Hermes to the Greeks) was the patron deity of Egyptian physicians. Imhotep also was deified after his death.

The religion of antiquity was conjoined with magic, and the belief was that illness was caused by evil spirits residing within the patient. These evil spirits could be the work of demons, or even of other persons who had control over such spirits, and it was the first job of the physician to determine the nature and source of the infecting spirit. He did this by interpreting omens. Bodily signs and symptoms often were taken as omens, but Babylonian physicians also examined the livers of sheep for divine direction in diagnosis. There were, in fact, three classes of physicians: the diviners, who foretold the course of the disease; the exorcists, who used incantations and other methods to drive out the evil spirit; and the physicians proper, who performed operations and administered drugs. The physician proper developed the practice of applying excrement and other obnoxious remedies to drive the demon from the unfortunate patient.

Many beliefs of the ancients left imprints on the practice of medicine that survive to this day. One such belief was that disease was beyond the control of the patient, and only through the magical power of the physician was there hope for recovery. It is noteworthy that the physician's role was not only sanctioned by society, but precisely demanded by a belief system that was largely directed by priests. Although our knowledge of ancient medicine is fragmentary and possibly inaccurate in some instances, the conclusion is inescapable that medicine did not emerge as an independent entity, but evolved indistinct from the social, cultural and religious practices of the time, and consistently reflected all aspects of society. The practices of physicians were determined not by their knowledge of biology, but by their personal and cultural beliefs. Their allegiance was primarily to the gods and only secondarily to sick mortals.

The awe of the patient, however, could not help but be directed to the physician as well as to the gods. Indeed, deification, as happened with Imhotep, was a natural consequence for those who did the work of the gods. Although early physicians used both religious and rational approaches to medicine, in the minds of the laity their power came from the gods, a notion that profoundly influenced the practice of medicine.

The Egyptians were the first to practice empirical medicine, a trial and error method that remains entrenched in modern medical practices. In the course of applying many remedies of diverse origins, physicians observed that some more than others were associated with a beneficial effect. These observations, often inaccurate and always tied to the general belief in the will of the gods as the source of healing, were nevertheless the basis for the first pharmacopoeia with rational roots,[1] the first alternative to supernatural medicine. The sacred books of Hermes, which contained the pharmacopoeia, were perhaps the first gift to posterity of a large body of medical knowledge.

There is one other characteristic of ancient medicine that merits mention. As long as the physician acted as an agent of the gods, a calamitous result for the patient was an act of the gods, despite the valiant intercession of the physician. If, however, the patient recovered, the physician was in a position to take credit, for would not the patient have died without his intervention? It is one of the more lasting peculiarities of the human psyche that, within a system of thought in which sickness is believed due to causes beyond the patient's control, if the patient recovers, the

1. Native herbal medicine in many parts of the world may have included drugs of some biological benefit, but their use would have been based on their presumed influence with the spirits rather than on rational observation of their benefit.

doctor gets the credit; if the patient dies, it is the fault of an external force. So long as the physician of antiquity operated within the belief system, the chance episodes of life and death made it appear that he had a positive power over illness.

Remedies, the means through which the physician interceded with the gods, were given similar credit. From what we know of disease, it is impossible to conclude other than that the foreboding array of animal feces and other foul substances used to drive away the evil spirits could only have produced disease, not cured it. But these remedies were believed to be essential to exorcism, and any harm they did was taken as a sign of the virulence of the offending spirit. Society accepted the practices, and physicians, who were after all servants of society, were as unaware as anyone else that their therapies were harmful, a situation that has its modern counterpart.

THE GREEK CONNECTION

In medicine as in almost every endeavor of Western civilization, the Greeks were the most influential source of our thinking. Their fundamental influence on Western medicine is seen in the deference given to the Hippocratic tradition and to the Hippocratic Oath, which was until recent years uttered by every graduating medical student.

Aesculapius[2] was the Greek god-equivalent of Imhotep. The myth of Aesculapius[3] has it that there lived in Thessaly, in northeast Greece, a maiden named Coronis, who was so beautiful that when the god Apollo surprised her bathing, he possessed her and made her pregnant. Afterward, when Coronis consented to her father's wish that she marry her cousin Ischus, Apollo (the god of light and truth) was angry to be so deceived. The result of his wrath was that Coronis was slain, either by Apollo himself or by one of the arrows of Artemis.

2. The Greek name is *Asklepios,* but the Latin *Aesculapius* is more commonly used.
3. Edith Hamilton, *Mythology,* pp. 279-81.

Then Apollo, contemplating the dead Coronis on the funeral pyre, assuaged his grief by plucking the almost-born Aesculapius from his mother's womb. He took the child to the cave of Chiron, the Centaur, who raised him.

Chiron knew much about the use of herbs, potions and incantations, and the young Aesculapius soon surpassed him in his ability to cure illness. Said to be often accompanied by a serpent, Aesculapius became a great physician and was much sought after. The news of his ability to cure spread across the land, and he was much honored among mortals. Votive tablets appeared telling of the miraculous healings. A woman from Athens, blind in one eye, went to Aesculapius, who slit open the eye and rubbed in balsam. Thereafter the patient could see perfectly well through both eyes. Others were cured of headaches and suppurating wounds, and the fame of Aesculapius was great.

But in the end Aesculapius drew down upon himself the anger of the gods by committing the greatest sin of a mortal, the assumption of godly powers. He dared to raise Hippolytus from the dead, a transgression that stirred the ire of Pluto, who complained that Hades was being depopulated. Zeus would not allow a mortal to have power over the dead, and he struck down Aesculapius with a thunderbolt, reinforcing the belief among mortals that healing was an act of the gods. After his death, temples arose to the cult of Aesculapius. These temples were run by priests who claimed to be descendants of the gods, and to have exclusive access to their healing powers, so that no self-styled practitioner might lay claim to being a healer.

The meaning of the myth of Aesculapius is clear: Healing is the domain of the gods, and man transgresses by not keeping his place in this function. This belief is still widely held, even in Western societies. Although the Egyptians and Mesopotamians developed some elements of what we might call rational medicine, the rational elements were not truly secular, as they were applied only within a religious context. The magical part of the cure remained its most important ingredient. One can only speculate that during the height of inquiry in ancient Egypt and Mesopotamia there were physicians on the fringe of conventional belief who stretched religious thought to accommodate their observations of natural phenomena. But the essence of mythology and magic is that new observations must be interpreted to fit old myths. The integrity of a culture often depends on doing this.

THE GREEK PHYSICIANS

The greatest contribution of the Greeks was the development of a systematic school of rational medicine. They were the first to rise above animism (belief in spirits) in their conception of disease, thereupon opening the way to rational therapy and scientific practices. One can not overestimate the importance of this break with the religio-magical system in influencing the course of Western medicine. Most certainly the break was not sudden, nor was it permanent or complete. Just as the Egyptians were able to practice empirical and magical medicine side by side, so were the Greeks. The rational emerged slowly, rising and ebbing according to circumstances. Just when this process began we do not know. But we do know that freedom of inquiry in Greek society allowed expression of rational thought that had not been possible in previous civilizations, and a second system of medicine grew up beside the older order.

The two systems of Greek medicine were the temples of the cult of Aesculapius and the secular school of medicine that evolved from them. Students of the latter, called the Aesculapiads, were the true physicians in today's sense, although they were not pure in their application of rational techniques, any more than the cultists were devoid of rationality, and there was occasionally overlapping of the two schools. I do not wish to imply that one school was run by charlatans who left us a legacy of superstition and irrational practices, whereas the other practiced totally scientific medicine, but there was a true distinction between the schools, allowing for the almost imperceptible emergence of methods that set the course of modern Western medicine.

The Aesculapiads are best known by the greatest of all physicians, Hippocrates. Very little is known in fact about Hippocrates. He was born on the island of Cos about 460 B.C., and he died sometime between 377 and 359. If the later date is correct, he lived to be 101 years old, appropriate enough for a great physician.[4] He was last heard of in Thessaly, the birthplace of Aesculapius, after a lifetime of wandering, teaching, and practicing medicine.

That Hippocrates did exist is attested by his contemporary Plato, who mentioned him respectfully, and by numerous writings that make reference to him. The ideal of the man represents the highest attainment of physicians in service to their patients. As is true of the deified doctors that preceded him, it is the image of Hippocrates more than his vaguely known deeds that leads physicians to aspire to godlike efforts. Very likely, those who followed him, and we ourselves, attribute to this man more than mortal qualities, but lack of factual detail allows a greater sense of what we think were his ideals. Calm and dignified, Hippocrates had a singleness of purpose: to benefit his patient even if it meant sacrificing himself. Observant, reflective, humble and comforting, he absorbed the agony of his patient's despair even when others withdrew, never deceiving, but giving meaning and dignity to suffering and death. He observed carefully and without distorting his observations for personal gain, teaching and learning from other physicians and those they served. At once knowing the limits of his own knowledge and ability, he taught by example that these limits are not fixed but must be respected. Humane, incorruptible, devoted to those he served, he was the ideal physician, a lasting inspiration to his profession.

The Hippocratic Corpus is a set of about seventy treatises

4. Henry E. Sigerist, *The Great Doctors*, p. 32; John Camp, *The Healer's Art*, pp. 29-30; Charles Singer and Ashworth E. Underwood, *A Short History of Medicine*, p. 28.

collected over the three or four centuries following the death of
Hippocrates, most of them presumably written by his pupils, or
by even later physicians following in his school.[5] That they are
not the work of one or a few authors writing in concert is evident
from the inconsistencies from book to book, including direct
contradictions. Even so, they are all in accord with the Hippocratic ideal, and a remarkable unity of purpose is found in
them. The ideas and methods described in the Corpus are not
altogether original, as the Greeks owed much to the civilizations that preceded them and were much influenced by the
mythology of their ancestors, the Egyptian and Mesopotamian
societies, the Sicilian, Athenian and Alexandrian schools, and
even Indian and Persian elements. A distillate of these diverse
sources was combined with learning from the Hippocratic
schools of Cos to make up this most important treatise in the
history of medicine.

There are three central hypotheses in the Hippocratic Corpus:
(1) all illness is due to some bodily malfunction, (2) the environment of the patient must be closely studied to arrive at a satisfactory diagnosis and prognosis, and (3) our own natures are the
physicians of our illnesses.[6] In practice, these principles were no
doubt unrefined and went hand-in-hand with the usual magical
rites, but the revolutionary change that the Hippocratic hypotheses put in motion loosened the grip of magic on medicine by
undermining the belief that illness is due to the imposition of
gods and demons with the notion that it is due to malfunction of
the body. This fundamental change in attitude allowed doctors
to look for causes and cures in the workings of nature. Disease
as the will of the gods was as fixed as the gods themselves, but
its manifestation in the human body became open to human
inquiry.

The Hippocratic school taught that health was maintained by
a harmonious balance of the four humors: blood (from the heart),

5. Singer and Underwood, *A Short History of Medicine*, pp. 22, 27.
6. Camp, *The Healer's Art*, pp. 33-34.

phlegm (from the brain), yellow bile (from the liver), and black bile (from the spleen).[7] An imbalance of these four humors caused disease—an excess of one bringing on a certain disease, and a deficiency of another resulting in some other malady. The Hippocratic physicians made much of these humors, suggesting that various body types and constitutions were associated with specific imbalances and that the human temperaments (i.e., the sanguine, the phlegmatic, the choleric, and the melancholic) were set according to the prevailing humor.

Lacking molecular chemistry, the Greeks retained a primitive notion of disease, but that they possessed the hubris to challenge its presumed supernatural origin[8] is what is important. The second Hippocratic hypothesis, that the environment of the patient must be studied to arrive at a satisfactory diagnosis and prognosis, supports the concept that disease, arising within the body, is of natural, not supernatural, origin. If disease is the will of the gods, one goes to the temple, but if it arises within the body, one looks around the body. The art of medicine thus became less spiritual; it became rational, which is to say that it was based on observation of natural phenomena. The Hippocratic physicians learned from all sources available, and by different methods, always keeping careful records, noting the infinite variety of experiences and cautiously drawing inferences from their limited knowledge and data. This approach was the

7. Bernard Dixon, *Beyond the Magic Bullet*, p. 7. This conception of disease was derived from primitive beliefs that attributed illness to imbalances that caused disharmony between man and the gods. The Greek adaptation of this idea was that imbalances caused disharmony between man and nature, a conception that placed disease within the realm of natural laws and produced what would become an enduring conflict between supernatural and natural schools of thought.

8. An exception was epilepsy, which the Greeks called "the Sacred Disease." To this Hippocrates answered: "It is thus with regard to the disease called Sacred: it appears to me to be nowise more divine nor more sacred than other diseases, but has a natural cause from which it originates like other affections. Men regard its nature and cause as divine from ignorance and wonder, because it is not at all like to other diseases." (*The Genuine Works of Hippocrates*, trans. Francis Adams, vol. 2, p. 334.)

forerunner of the modern scientific method. Perhaps the greatest clinical achievement of the Hippocratic books is the fine descriptions of individual cases. They are clear and succinct, objective and nonjudgmental. They record the facts rather than editorializing about the skills of the attending physicians. As examples of medical observations, they remain an excellent model for clinical records.

The third Hippocratic hypothesis, that our own natures are the physicians of our illnesses, arose from the new concept of bodily disease. Cures that previously had been credited to the gods were now perceived as coming from the body itself, or from nature. Thus, the "healing power of nature" became the first line of therapy. Observing that most patients recovered without any therapy, the Hippocratic physicians became reluctant to interfere with the natural process by applying medicinals of unknown benefit. They did not hesitate to use the knife when necessary, or to employ one of their limited number of drugs, but they were often content to wait on nature and did not intervene unless nature was failing. There was much that they could do, however, to assist nature, with diet, nursing, and exercise. They understood the importance of the healing milieu, as we see in this statement attributed to Hippocrates: "Not only should the doctor be ready to do his duty, but the patient, the assistants, and external circumstances must conspire to effect a cure."[9] How different from leaving it all to the gods!

Hippocrates laid out the path from superstition to science. Since his time medicine has been a blend of the natural and the supernatural. I intend to show that the supernatural still predominates in medicine and is the source of the profession's modern inadequacies and limitations. But the teachings of Hippocrates made the scientific method in medicine possible from his time onward.

Aristotle, 384-322 B.C., pupil of Plato and tutor of Alexander, changed the direction of medicine after Hippocrates and left his

9. Dixon, *Beyond the Magic Bullet*, p. 7.

permanent stamp on science.[10] Known primarily as a
philosopher, he was also the first great biologist, the founder of
comparative anatomy, and a writer of botanical books that are
still read today. He gave us what may have been the first anatom-
ical sketches, and he was the great codifier in all areas of science.
An observant naturalist, he actually described human evolution,
although he did not articulate the concept. In his influence on
medical thought he is best known for his errors: He believed that
the heart was the seat of intelligence, and he made no distinction
between arteries and veins. He held the ancients' theory that
there were four fundamental qualities —the hot and the cold, the
wet and the dry—and linked them with the four elements that
constitute living matter: earth, air, fire and water. Although his
true accomplishments were his discoveries and classifications
of botanical and anatomic structures, what later students revered most were his fallacious theories and syllogisms. His
doctrine of the four elements persisted in its entirety until the
seventeenth century, and it remains one of the great ironies of
medical history that a man whose observations and records were
among the finest of all time should deed to posterity a methodology based more on philosophical theory than on observation and
experience.

The man who brought Greek creative science to an end was
Galen (A.D. 131-200). Caught in the converging streams of the
Hippocratic method and Aristotelian thought,[11] Galen drowned
the substance of the Hippocratic Corpus in Aristotelian form.
Galen's thinking was deterministic. He reverted to the pre-
Hippocratic notion that all things were determined by forces
outside man. The Creator, the omniscient God, made man the
reflection of His perfection, a point of view agreeable to the then
emerging Christianity. Galen claimed a complete knowledge of
the laws of God and nature that few have ever dared to presume.

10. Singer and Underwood, *A Short History of Medicine*, pp. 41-47.
11. Ibid., pp. 59-67; Sigerist, *The Great Doctors*, p. 68; Camp, *The Healer's Art*,
pp. 42-43.

Gone was the humble, cautious Hippocratic search for knowledge, replaced by contentiousness, pedantry and arrogance. The lofty idealism of the Greeks who went to their patients seeking knowledge gave way to self-satisfaction and blunted inquiry. The writings of Galen, in more or less adulterated form, provided the theoretical basis of medical practice for the next fifteen hundred years. Although Galen was able to divert medicine from the scientific track Hippocrates had set it on, the two great contributions of the Greeks — the ideal of the humane physician, and the methodology of the Hippocratic school — would not remain suppressible.

MEDIEVAL MEDICINE

Whereas the Galenic writings found favor with Christianity and with Islam because of obeisance to the supremacy of God, the doctrines of Christianity and Greek science were inherently opposed. To the new faith, the source of healing was God, and pagan physicians who espoused rational explanations of disease and healing were unacceptable to the church. Christ was the Great Healer, and in the struggle for the allegiance of minds the miracles of Christ vied with the cures of the Greeks. This conflict undoubtedly had many battlegrounds, not the least important of which was social policy. The aristocratic Greeks held that health and medical care were privileges of the rich and noble, while the Christians taught salvation of all sinners, and promoted the concept of medical care for all the sick. The choice, in simplistic terms, was between rational medicine for the few and spiritual medicine for the many. With the ascendancy of Christianity, Greek medicine was eclipsed by the church.

The function of healing having become the prerogative of the church, secular physicians became fewer. Gradually physicians became clerics, or perhaps it was the other way around, but the principle that healing should be accessible to all the sick meant that during the Dark Ages most of medicine was under the control of the church. It was then that the writings of Galen and

Avicenna, the systematist of Arabian medicine, dominated medical thinking. As the history of medicine has been inseparable from that of the rest of society, however, the Renaissance restored to medicine some of the advances of the early Greeks and set it back on the path to science.

THE ADVENT OF SCIENTIFIC MEDICINE

Since my purpose in recounting this medical history is to show the philosophic progression of medicine, I need mention only a few of the many persons who brought it out of the Dark Ages. Perhaps the most outstanding was Vesalius (1514-64), the great anatomist and surgeon. To summarize this man's epoch-making contribution: he questioned the theories of Aristotle and Galen, and found that the statements of the latter in particular were not borne out by his own observations of anatomy. His reliance on dissection and rigorous observation destroyed forever the medieval theories of the structure and function of the human body. The work of Vesalius, perhaps more than any other, re-aimed medicine in the scientific direction from which it had been so long turned away.

Paracelsus, contemporary of Vesalius, was an alchemist known as the King of the Quacks. For all his mistaken theories and arrogance, he was to leave his mark by rejecting Galen and insisting on observation and experience in the practice of medicine. There followed the contributions, among many, of Paré, Harvey, Malpighi, Syndenham, Hunter, Jenner, Laennec, Bernard, Virchow, Pasteur, Koch and Lister, all names known to every medical student.

This is not to imply that from the time of Vesalius there was a complete triumph of enlightenment over darkness, of science over superstition. The actual practice of medicine remained predominantly empirical, an amalgam of magic, custom and social beliefs. But from then on, the pursuit of science was possible, and indeed it became the dominant theoretical concept in the development of Western medicine. The proportion of superstition and science in medicine since then has been adjusted by the personal, cultural and professional beliefs of the physicians who choose between them.

The lessons of the history of medicine are that in all ages practices of physicians have mirrored the beliefs of the community, and — however much they were intended to help patients — they have been based more on social policies than on a detached assessment of benefit to patients. In our later examination of modern medical practices, we shall see that they are remarkably like those of the ancient physicians.

CHAPTER TWO

Why People Go to Doctors

A desire to take medicine is perhaps the great feature which distinguishes man from other animals.

William Osler

SOCIAL NECESSITY

JUST AS societies have always needed politicians to deal with political matters, and priests to answer religious questions, they have required doctors to give meaning to sickness and to explain the relationship of disease to cosmology and existence, and the relationship of the sick to the rest of society. Perhaps the first specialist when man began to think was the shaman, who combined the offices of priest and physician.

The most frightening and intolerable condition of sickness is to have no explanation of the cause, as this means not knowing how bad the illness is, how long it will last, how to combat it, and whether it is contagious. The first important function of the physician has always been to explain the illness within the context of religious or cosmic beliefs so that the patient can deal with it emotionally and the community can deal with it socially.

Every culture has had its own conception of the origin of disease. It doesn't matter that explanations have varied from time to time, or from culture to culture, or that a particular belief was physiologically or anatomically inaccurate. If a shaman told a patient that his illness was caused by a particular evil spirit, and this made sense to the patient and the community, the shaman fulfilled a social need, even before he began his treatment, by giving legitimacy to the sickness. The shaman provided a service to the surrounding community, since if a person was possessed by a devil, it was in the community interest to find out.

The modern physician serves society in much the same way, by explaining the behavior of its members, by sanctioning some deviant behavior as legitimate illness, and by setting the rules of conduct for sick people and those with whom they interact. Today, if a man becomes unable to perform his job properly because of chest pain with physical activity, the physician confirms the patient's status as an ill person in a way that the patient himself can not. His employer requires him to see a physician not so much out of a humanitarian desire to provide care, but so as to maintain a consistent social policy regarding illness and work among employees. Even if the physician makes an incorrect diagnosis, society's demands for an explanation it recognizes as authoritative are fulfilled.

THE BELIEF THAT DOCTORS CAN CURE

> For everybody's family doctor was remarkably clever, and was understood to have immeasurable skill in the management and treatment of the most skittish or vicious diseases. The evidence of his cleverness was of the higher intuitive order, lying in his lady patients' immovable conviction, and was unassailable by any objection.
>
> George Eliot,
> *Middlemarch*

> The efficient physician is the man who successfully amuses his patients while nature effects a cure.
>
> Voltaire

One fact is indisputable about physicians: Historically, they have been exceedingly successful. To be sure, they have had failures, and there have been periods when as a class they were unpopular—as during the Dark Ages, when clerics preempted their function—but throughout most of history the services of doctors have been sought fervently and desperately. Looking at early medical practices, one finds it difficult to account for such success.

Until about two centuries ago, doctors could give little more than moral or psychosomatic help, minor amelioration of pain as with opiates, help with trauma, and quarantine,[1] and the inescapable conclusion is that they did much harm. It makes one recoil to think of applying animal excrement or boiling oil to open wounds and blowing septic materials down throats or other orifices. Practices that could not possibly correct an anatomic or physiologic abnormality—cupping, bleeding, purging and inducing vomiting—could only have weakened a person who was already sick. But the remarkable thing is that these treatments were not perceived as harmful by either patient or physician or society. People flocked to receive these treatments.

Until fifty years ago when sulfa, the first of the antibiotics, was discovered, doctors knew of no drug that would kill infectious bacteria. They used herbal medicines to relieve symptoms, performed limited surgery and midwifery, set broken bones, and injected vaccines to stop the spread of disease, but they had almost no means to cure a disease. Nevertheless, people have always gone to doctors, believed in doctors, and attributed to doctors the fact that they got well. To understand this we need to understand two concepts: (1) the body's natural recovery mechanisms, and (2) psychological influences on healing.

THE HEALING POWER OF NATURE

It is estimated that seventy to eighty percent of the people who go to doctors have nothing wrong with them that wouldn't be

1. Richard H. Shryock, *Medicine in America*, p. 5.

cleared up by a vacation, a pay raise, or relief from everyday emotional stress. Only ten percent require drugs or surgery to get well, and approximately ten percent have diseases for which there is no known cure.

The first secret of the doctor's success has always been that most ill persons get well through the natural recovery mechanisms of the body, without which even the fittest would not have survived. The Hippocritic physicians called it the "healing power of nature," and a later phrase for it was *vis medicatrix naturae* ("the body's ability to heal itself"). But once the patient was in the hands of the doctor, all subsequent recoveries were attributed to him, regardless of what the natural course of events would have been. The built-in natural success rate of over eighty percent recovery from all illnesses, when credited to the doctor, was enough to guarantee accolades to the profession notwithstanding the fate of the remaining twenty percent.

Most people do not realize that most illnesses run a benign course, with eventual recovery. Physicians mistakenly attach a worse prognosis to illnesses left untreated than is warranted, thereby creating the illusion of successful "treatment." Illnesses that run their course to disability or death within a short period of time have always been few compared to all illnesses. Therefore, if a doctor, or a specific type of treatment, was associated with an illness, the healer or the remedy was given the credit for healing that would have occurred naturally. This was the primary process by which doctors were "successful" even when they had no remedies of true benefit.

A related work of nature doctors get credit for involves spontaneous changes in chronic conditions. The classic example is rheumatoid arthritis, which may on occasion disappear altogether; but usually the symptoms and the physical disability come and go. Spontaneous changes, for better or worse, are an invariable characteristic of this disease, which has an unpredictable course. Failure to understand that approximately a third of patients are likely to improve no matter what the treatment, and that almost all patients will have periods of improvement if you wait long enough, results in a false imputation of healing power to the doctor.[2]

In chronic illnesses, extreme conditions regress toward a less extreme state. Patients who have long-standing illnesses tend to see their doctors during these extremes, and particularly during the worst periods. If a patient goes to the doctor when the symptoms are at their worst, it follows that he will usually get better soon afterwards. If there were a rule that patients with chronic illnesses could see the doctor only on one day of the week, or on a particular day of the month, regardless of how well they felt, they would be as likely to get worse as to get better after the medical encounter. If these patients went to physicians only when their chronic illnesses were not causing problems, they would undoubtedly notice a tendency to feel worse afterwards.

Not understanding natural healing phenomena, both patient and doctor mistakenly credit the doctor and his treatment with the cure. Imagine the reaction of a physician five thousand years ago when, after he had administered a remedy for a condition believed to be fatal, the patient recovered. It was natural for the physician to believe that he did have curing power. This classic error, post hoc, ergo propter hoc ("after this, therefore because of this") is the primordial professional experience of the doctor, repeated by every physician and healer who ever practiced. The concept was disputed by the Hippocratic physicians but allowed to flourish again after their fall. Post hoc, ergo propter hoc is not, however, applied to medical failures, which are attributed to causes beyond the physician's power today as they were in antiquity. Successful results have the effect of reinforcing medical beliefs; unsuccessful results do not produce any questioning.

Further supporting the fallacy is the natural tendency of doc-

2. I once heard a professor in medical school say that injections of gold are effective in the treatment of rheumatoid arthritis, particularly when given shortly before a spontaneous remission. He said this with a straight face.

tors to remember successful cases and forget unsuccessful ones. Cures have always been widely advertised, while failures with the same treatment went unnoticed or were soon forgotten, and the remedy was regarded as beneficial on the strength of apparent successes. Especially in times when there were no real means of opposing mysterious and often fatal diseases, it was important to the community to believe in the curative power of the healer. Thus, as with Aesculapius, reports of cures were widely spread and became part of the lore, whereas obvious failures were quickly forgotten.

The doctor's interest in the success of the treatment was matched by that of the patient. It was a symbiotic relationship in which the wishes of one fulfilled those of the other: The reassurance of the doctor produced improvement in the patient that in turn was evidence to both of the correctness of the doctor's ministrations. This reciprocal belief-building was further enhanced by elimination of negative feedback: When the result was negative, the patient either died or did not return. The process was (and still is) little understood by either, and with good reason—to see it as mutual delusion would be self-defeating for both. There was, then, complicity between patient and doctor to help each other fulfill their desires to be well, on the one hand, and to make well, on the other. This complicity was the cornerstone of mutual belief in worthless remedies. It in no way, however, invalidated the true compassion of the physician or the patient's appreciative response.

Even the most forceful physician or witch doctor could not have relied solely upon his words or claimed powers as instruments of healing. Almost from the beginning, physicians developed remedies and procedures through which they healed, and which kept them apart from the ordinary man who did not possess these necessary tools. Perhaps the first medium of therapy was the rattle. Herbs, drugs and other ingestants were not far behind, as we know from the earliest medical records. Surgery also was used almost from the beginning, along with various ceremonial incantations, exorcisms, and other forms of what today we would call psychotherapy. The most popular medium today is complex technology.

One can, then, from the inception of the practice of medicine, recognize two parts to the therapeutic process: the doctor and his relationship to the patient, and the therapeutic media. Although the therapies and procedures are what patients and historians notice, and what most characterize the practice of medicine in the minds of the public, they are in reality the smaller part of the therapeutic process.

PSYCHOLOGICAL INFLUENCES ON HEALING

Psychological phenomena have always contributed to the success of doctors in relieving symptoms—making the patient feel better—and in actually promoting recovery from specific diseases by enhancing natural healing. Sufferers who went to the Aesculapian temples spent several days in psychological preparation—undergoing fasting, fumigations, purgations, baths, and other purification rites—before beginning the curing ceremonies.[3] During this time they daily scanned the votive tablets that recorded the miraculous healings of Aesculapius. In this setting of extreme tension and expectation, some patients were relieved of their ills prior to the ultimate ceremony.[4]

When spiritual preparation had reached its zenith, the patient was conducted into the holiest sanctuary, where he made an offering before the gold and ivory image of Aesculapius. By then in a well-orchestrated trance of belief, he was induced to lie down to sleep within the courts, where Aesculapius, attended by his daughter, the goddess Hygieia, and a serpent, would appear in a dream. The god passed by each patient, performing the task necessary to cure him. The lame walked, the deaf could hear the singing of the birds, pain was gone, and wounds were

3. Henry E. Sigerist, *The Great Doctors*, p. 25.
4. A modern analogy is the patient with asthma, who, extremely apprehensive and gasping for breath during an acute attack, begins to breathe more easily as soon as the doctor arrives, even before receiving medication.

healed. The grateful patients gave offerings and thanks, leaving the inner courts of the temple as living testimony to the healing force that awaited those outside. What made these patients, who had received no actual curative therapy in the modern sense, get better?

The mechanisms by which psychological factors influence healing are complex and incompletely understood, but their effects are profound and universal. For example, in coronary artery disease, the common form of heart disease, it is recognized that adverse emotional factors can increase chest pain and accelerate and worsen the physical disease. Anxiety and despair can be fatal, but expectation and hope are therapeutic. Any physician knows that any procedure, treatment, ceremony or statement that gives hope will cause marked symptomatic improvement. Think of how you have reacted to news of a new treatment, or the promise of a trusted religious leader, that might help you or a loved one who is ill. Anyone who assumes the role of doctor, or shaman, automatically invokes hope in patients conditioned to expect help from him. Thus it is well known that a medical student can get the same short-term results as a physician if the patient thinks the student is the doctor.[5] Evidence of the healing power of faith has accumulated over the centuries, and doctors have always capitalized on it. From the beginning—from the rituals of magic to coronary bypass surgery—healers have been able to mobilize the natural healing resources by evoking in the patient hope, expectation of recovery, and confidence in the doctor's ability to cure.

A large part of the distress accompanying illness is due to uncertainty and to fear of what might happen. The mere presence of the doctor is often enough to relieve this apprehension and alleviate the symptoms. Pain, especially, is tied to apprehension, so that generally speaking, relief of apprehension will result in relief of pain. In fact, the patient with the most

5. Jerome D. Frank, *Persuasion and Healing*, p. 167.

apprehension and the most distress is the one who will improve the most when the apprehension is removed.

The success of doctors is in no small part due to their professional ability to comfort. Although friends and family also are capable of giving comfort—and their presence is important to an ill person—they share the patient's own beliefs and apprehensions too much to be as comforting as the doctor, who is experienced in dealing with distressed patients and is vested with the authority and power to take away the cause of distress. The doctor not only gives comfort by his words and deeds, but orchestrates and directs the comforting activities of those persons around the patient.

Without question, comforting promotes healing. Studies using modern techniques of psychological testing have shown that any procedure that convinces the patient of the doctor's interest and desire to help produces a striking and lasting relief of symptoms, even when the symptoms are due to specific diseases. Perhaps the crucial therapeutic element for the patient is knowing that the doctor cares and will help in any way possible.

Despair or grief is often a part of the genesis of a disease, and the person who is demoralized from an illness is less likely to recover, or will recover more slowly, than the person who is not demoralized. This is a clinical fact observed by all physicians and many laymen. Any kind of therapy that combats demoralization or produces positive changes of attitude—quiet talk, shaking rattles, or more sophisticated medical or surgical procedures—will counter distress and facilitate natural recovery from any patient who wants to get well. (The patient's desire to get well is a critical part of the process.) Although a good physician should be credited with using this resource, the true source of recovery is more often the patient's attitude toward his illness than any specific therapy.

The patient's response to the disease may be altered by suggestion. At all times, the patient makes an assessment of his illness by interpreting what he feels and what he is told. The interpretation is colored by what he thinks is causing illness or pain. Consider two patients who are suffering from headache because of brain tumor. If, without any real change in the size of tumor, the first patient receives a strong suggestion that it is increasing, he will likely report increased head pain, whereas if the second patient receives the suggestion that his tumor is shrinking, he will likely report a decrease in pain. Under hypnotic suggestion, ordinary pain sensations can be reduced and even totally blocked from consciousness. Suggestion can also induce actual physical changes.

It is commonplace to see a person with a functional disorder (an illness in which physical disorders can be influenced by attitude or emotion), markedly improve as the result of suggestion. Healing of ulcers, migraine headaches, skin rashes, life-threatening colitis, and other serious illnesses often follows strong suggestion by the therapist that the disorder is cured. There is nothing extraordinary or miraculous about this. It happens every day and can be duplicated by any physician or healer who understands the art of suggestion. Suggestion is used in Navaho healing ceremonies where patients are encouraged to develop images of the healing process. A modern adaptation is having cancer patients visualize cells attacking and shrinking their tumors. Biofeedback is the current technique for the age-old attempt to heal by controlling bodily functions with the mind.

How, we must ask, does suggestion work to alter bodily functions? How does the mind get in touch with the stomach? The intermediary is the nervous system.

There are actually two nervous systems, voluntary and involuntary (autonomic). Ordinarily, we have conscious control over the voluntary system but not over the involuntary system. The voluntary system regulates the muscles we use in our daily activities, such as walking, running, eating, talking and writing. The nerves of this system send signals to the muscles, and damage to the nerves results in loss of muscle function, as occurs with polio or injuries to the spinal cord. We can control these muscles as long as they are able to work normally. Occasionally we inflict damage upon them by running to exhaustion or wounding each other in fighting, but in general we use our voluntary nervous systems to protect ourselves and to maintain health.

Virtually all of the work of the involuntary system takes place through reflexes or automatic responses that we don't usually notice. This system regulates the functioning of the internal organs, such as the liver, heart, intestines, kidneys, and lungs. Breathing is largely an involuntary action, although we can augment it, or even override our normal breathing patterns for short periods of time if we want to. For the most part, though, we are not conscious of our breathing, because it is a reflexive response to the amount of oxygen in the blood and the amount of air in the lungs. There is constant feedback of information to let the breathing center in the nervous system know how much oxygen the blood needs to support the body's activity.

Unfortunately, the involuntary system can malfunction. If it stimulates too much acid secretion in the stomach, the result is an ulcer. If the blood vessels, which can open or constrict under the influence of the nervous system, are not set at the proper opening size, the result is a headache or high blood pressure or angina (heart pain). Asthma, a condition in which the small air tubes do not open widely enough, is to some degree a malfunction of the involuntary system, as are colitis, constipation and diarrhea, menstrual disorders, skin rashes and irregular heartbeats. These disorders may have other causes, but since the respective organs are regulated by the involuntary system, it can initiate the disorder or compensate for it. For instance, even though in some persons asthma may not be caused by a malfunction of the involuntary system, any successful treatment must modify the nerve reflexes enough to make them open the small airways.

The involuntary nervous system is influenced by the emotions. Anxiety, anger, fear, depression and virtually all strong negative emotions upset the involuntary system and produce changes in the functioning of the internal organs. Any physician knows that the high-powered businessman, or the person always working under pressure, is the one most likely to have an ulcer or a heart attack. Scientific studies have shown that changes of emotion change the rate of acid secretion in the stomach, blood pressure, the cross-sectional size of arteries, movement of the intestines, and heart rate. Some emotions release powerful natural therapeutic chemicals, such as cortisone, thyroid and endorphins, into the blood stream.[6] If anxiety increases acid secretions in the stomach, tranquility reduces them. Suggestion, by the shaman or physician, that the source of the disease is eliminated may not only bring peace of mind, but may stimulate positive emotions causing physical changes in the internal organs that will induce healing.

These changes may be transient—in fact, they are usually difficult to sustain by words alone—but they are nonetheless therapeutic. They make the internal environment favorable to healing and accelerate the normal healing processes. This is, of course, the object of all therapy. Through the ages charisma has played an important part in the doctor's ability to heal. Doctors with forceful personalities have been able to cure or ameliorate disorders by telling patients that they are going to get well.

The Placebo Effect

Suggestion can be spoken or implied. By the very act of giving medicine or treatment, the doctor implies that the therapy will remove the cause of the illness. If the doctor believes the illness is untreatable with medicine, he may nevertheless prescribe

6. One study was made in a hospital whose policy prohibited the presence of family or friends with women in labor. Women who were assigned a supportive woman companion during labor had a markedly decreased complication rate and an average labor period ten hours shorter than women who did not have a companion. (R. Sosa et al., "The Effect of a Supportive Companion on Perinatal Problems, Length of Labor, and Mother-Infant Interaction," *New England Journal of Medicine* 303(1980):597-600.)

something so that the patient can get the benefits of the therapeutic suggestion. Such a prescription is called a *placebo*.

In Latin the verb *placebo* means "I shall please," and so a placebo, literally, is any therapeutic substance or procedure that pleases the patient. In modern usage, however, a placebo is most often a therapy (usually a pill or injection) that the doctor thinks is biologically worthless but harmless. If a patient asks for a pain pill or a tranquilizer, for example, the doctor may prescribe a sugar pill, which he believes will nevertheless please the patient who thinks he is receiving effective medicine. Placebos have a bad name with doctors and patients alike, but some doctors give placebos without realizing it. Take, for instance, the use of sulfur by alchemists. Paracelsus, the alchemist physician, believed strongly in the beneficial effects of sulfur, and when he prescribed it, he was unaware that it was nothing more than a placebo. He thought it could cure under the proper circumstances. We now think, from our knowledge of sulfur, that it was worthless and even harmful as used by Paracelsus. Yet his patients reported improvement from the drug, believing that it made them better.

An important distinction is that the drug was not given as a placebo. In other words, a drug or treatment need not be thought of as a placebo by the doctor in order to produce the *placebo effect*, which is the positive reaction of the patient to a treatment, quite aside from its biological benefit.[7]

If a person believes that any treatment is beneficial, he will react positively to that treatment. The placebo effect is as old as therapy itself. Patients with chest pain due to heart disease (angina), will consistently report a decreased amount and severity of the pain when given any therapy that they think is effective. This does not mean that placebos work as well as drugs that go directly to the source of pain, but it does show that pain can be reduced when the patient believes the treatment is working.

In a very real way, the placebo effect is an extension of the

7. Thomas A. Preston, *Coronary Artery Surgery*, pp. 81-98.

healing power of the physician, because it is the physician's use of the treatment that imbues it with curative powers. Physicians with patients being readied for coronary bypass surgery have observed a dramatic example of the placebo effect. Bypass surgery must be preceded by a diagnostic test (coronary angiography), which is actually a minor operation. During the test, tubes are inserted into the heart from incisions in the skin, and the patient is aware of physicians working on his heart. Occasionally, a patient mistakes this test for the bypass operation, especially if there is some discomfort during the procedure. Following the test such patients have reported absence of symptoms and a return of strength and health. Such cures have persisted for days or weeks until the patient discovered his error.

Further evidence of psychological influences on healing is coming from investigations into the nature of pain. Recent research suggests that enkephalin and endorphin, morphinelike peptides found naturally in the brain, inhibit pain.[8] These substances seem to be regulated by psychological factors, including stress,[9] and there is evidence linking the analgesic effect of placebos to release by the brain of these natural drugs,[10] although there is as yet no conclusive proof of a cause and effect relationship.

As the great North American physician Osler said about eighty years ago, "A desire to take medicine is perhaps the great feature which distinguishes man from other animals." The historical success of medicine depends in large part on this feature. The physicians of all times have maintained their honored positions and reputations as healers through inadvertent reliance on the placebo effect, without which most treatments would have been of no value.

8. N.I.H. Conference, "Basic and Clinical Studies of Endorphins," *Annals of Internal Medicine* 91(1979):239-50.

9. Ibid.; Editorial, *Lancet* 2(1978):819-20.

10. J.D. Levine, N.C. Gordon and H.L. Fields, "The Mechanism of Placebo Anesthesia," *Lancet* 2(1978):654-57.

THE STATUS OF PHYSICIANS

With notable exceptions, physicians have historically held a privileged if not exalted position within society. The Romans, for instance, made the Greek slave physicians freemen, as well as exempting them from taxes and military duty. For most of history the personal advantage of the physician has been social rather than economic. Until as late as the last century it was not at all unusual for a physician to be poor despite his hard work. It is only in recent years that wealth for physicians has been guaranteed by many societies through "social" legislation.

The special status of the physician strengthened, as well as grew from, professional exclusivity. If anyone with minimal experience had been permitted to perform the therapeutic ceremony, the physician's claim to special powers, and hence to special status, would have been undermined. The Aesculapian Greek physicians guarded their exclusivity by allowing only ordained members of the temple to perform healing rites, and these members were selected by the presiding group. Special access to the gods provided an embargo against entrance into the group by outsiders, thereby creating a certain professional aloofness from the surrounding society. When divine association weakened as a source of professional exclusivity — after medical practice was transferred from the church back to the secular realm — the usual guild and social means of maintaining control over entrance into a profession took its place. Today it is possible more than ever before for qualified students to enter medical school without previous professional associations, but until very recently admissions to the medical guild were regulated by professional and social means.

Part and parcel of professional autonomy, which grew out of exclusivity and the social need for the physician to be different, was absence of public scrutiny of medical practices. Since the physician was thought to have extraordinary powers not available to the public, the nonphysician was not in a position to question the logic or actions of the physician. There were exceptions to this rule, such as the harsh penalties for erring physicians enacted under the Code of Hammurabi (penalties which were, however, seldom assessed), but in general those who lacked the expertise or authority of the physician were powerless to challenge him. Physicians, for their part, encouraged their own authority and autonomy by not discussing professional methods or rationale with nonphysicians and by impressing upon physician trainees that they must not share professional methods or secrets with patients.

The physician, then, has maintained high status over the ages by fulfilling important social needs and by capitalizing on natural healing. All societies have needed physicians to explain disease, intercede with the presumed forces of disease, and give meaning to the interrelationship of life, illness, death and the surrounding world.

CHAPTER THREE

Physicians, Quacks and Healers

> Doctoring is not even the art of keeping people in health (no doctor seems able to advise you what to eat any better than his grandmother or the nearest quack); it is the art of curing illnesses.
>
> George Bernard Shaw
> *The Doctor's Dilemma*

KINDS OF DOCTORS

IN NORTH America physicians are doctors who hold the M.D. degree.[1] They make up the orthodox medical profession and are descendants of the early doctors who dealt with natural phenomena—those who developed the ancient Egyptian pharmacopoeia, the Hippocratic physicians, the bone-setters, the barber surgeons. They are the rationalists, who base their practices on anatomic and pharmacologic knowledge.

There has always been rivalry between orthodox physicians and others whom we shall call healers. Both groups differ from quacks, who by definition practice deliberate deceit, although there is of course always overlap, with no practitioner being totally guileless and some quacks perhaps not being totally

---

1. There are exceptions to this. In many areas of North America, osteopaths have the same legal and professional standing as M.D.'s. In many other countries orthodox physicians do not generally have the M.D. degree, but have equivalent training. All graduates of conventional medical schools will be considered physicians in this discussion.

deceitful. The distinction between physician and healer has not always been clear, but one big difference is that physicians primarily treat diseases, whereas healers treat illnesses.

ILLNESS AND DISEASE: TWO DIFFERENT POINTS OF VIEW

> There was only one question Ivan Ilyich wanted answered: was his condition dangerous or not? But the doctor ignored that question as irrelevant. From the doctor's point of view, such a question was unworthy of consideration. One had only to weigh possibilities: floating kidneys, chronic catarrh, or an ailment of the caecum. There was no question of the life of Ivan Ilyich—nothing but a contest between floating kidneys and the caecum.
>
> Tolstoy,
> "The Death of Ivan Ilyich"

Since the advent of scientific methods of learning how the body works biologically, physicians have moved away from dealing with patients' symptoms toward working with the bodily malfunctions their tests and instruments show. Simply put, in modern usage *disease* is the biological disorder the doctor finds, whereas *illness* is the patient's experience of his problem. The two are often not the same. The patient whose X ray shows a duodenal ulcer but who has no symptoms to match has disease without illness. The patient with abdominal pain but no duodenal ulcer according to his X ray, has an illness but no detected disease. The patient's concern is the illness, regardless of cause; the physician looks for and treats disease.

A physician making rounds one day came across a young patient who had been admitted to the hospital because of a heart murmur. The patient felt perfectly well; she had no pain or disability. But after listening to the intern's discussion of the findings, which included the murmur and two minor laboratory abnormalities, the physician exclaimed, "This patient has three diseases!" That the patient had no illness was of little consequence to the physician, who was intent upon tracking clues to disease. Ultimately the heart murmur was deemed "innocent" (many murmurs are normal, especially in young people), but the bedside discussion of "disease" left the patient with anxiety over her condition, thereby creating for her an illness.

The same disease may cause totally different illnesses in different patients. One patient with a heart attack, fearing that he will be disabled for the rest of his life, may suffer a prolonged illness, while another patient with a heart attack of the same severity may disregard it and not even seek medical help. The second patient in effect has no illness. About eighty percent of people who go to doctors have illnesses that can not be accounted for by disease. On the other hand, many people have serious disease without symptoms (illness).

The illness/disease dichotomy has its parallel in therapy. To the modern physician, curing means eradicating disease, regardless of the effect on the patient's illness. Healing, on the other hand, is the alleviation of illness or enhancement of natural biological recovery, by psychological mechanisms. In everyday language we often use *healing* and *curing* interchangeably. For instance, we say a wound is *healed*, not *cured*, although recovery was a physical process. In order to distinguish between the physical and emotional (or interpretive) processes, I shall use *healing* to mean the latter.

Curing, as used in this book, implies elimination or alleviation of disease over and above what is possible through nonspecific natural healing. It means bringing about a measurable physical change. A person who has pneumonia confirmed by X ray and physical examination is cured when the physical signs of pneumonia disappear. A person whose leg has atrophied because of polio is cured when he regains use of the leg and the muscle size has returned to normal. A cure is the result of *specific* treatment, as pneumonia is cured by an antibiotic, other therapies being ineffective.

Healing, on the other hand, is undetectable by physical tests. It is an emotional state in the patient that may or may not coexist with a cure, and affects the body only through nonspecific interaction of mind and body. For instance, if a person feeling ill goes to a native healer and after a ceremony of dancing and chanting says he is no longer ill, he has been healed but may or may not have been cured. In fact, there is no way of knowing whether he had disease to start with. The entire process was interpretive and not physically measurable.

Healing is associated with fulfillment, what the ancients and modern healers speak of as a feeling of emotional harmony, or a sense of attunement to or unity with the surrounding world. It induces in the patient a feeling that there is a "rightness" or balance in his relationship to others, to nature, and to God. Healing is nonspecific in that it is not the direct result of a specific therapy, but it may be achieved by any nonspecific process that puts the psychological healing mechanisms in motion. The only requirement for successful healing, as in the case of the ancient physicians, is that the ceremony conform to the patient's beliefs.

QUACKS

> There is a class of minds much more ready to believe that which is at first sight incredible, and because it is incredible, than what is generally thought reasonable.
>
> Oliver Wendell Holmes

The history of quackery parallels the history of medicine, the techniques of quacks imitating established medical practice and constantly skirting its fringes. The medical profession, in fact, created the setting that makes quackery hard to detect. Superstitious faith in doctors, which has always been encouraged by the profession, opened the door to quacks and keeps it open.

The exploits of the bold quacks of history make exciting reading.[2] The ingenuity and daring of these individuals inspire admiration that borders on forgiveness until one realizes how they exploited and harmed their victims. One of the most famous of all quacks was the legendary John St. John Long of London,

2. James H. Young, *The Medical Messiahs.*

who practiced his art in the early 1880s.[3] Although not a bona fide physician, he set up a practice on Harley Street, the locale of London's most eminent medical practitioners. He gained a reputation for, among other things, treating tuberculosis by rubbing liniment into the patient's skin, which allegedly drew out the disease. The success of his fraudulent practice can be measured by his immense fortune and wide popularity as a healer. He was a quack because his liniment had no curative component and he knew it.

The difference between quacks and conventional doctors whose therapies fail to cure is largely a difference in intent. Sometimes the line between them becomes blurred, as I shall discuss later.

FORMS OF QUACKERY

Most quackery involves therapy. There can be quackery in diagnosis as well, but usually the fraudulent healer treats patients who think they already know what their trouble is. If a man selling snake oil to a crowd suggests that the liquid is capable of curing arthritis, the person who steps forward to make the purchase assumes responsibility for the diagnosis. The quack practitioner knows that people pay money to get well, and that in most cases even grandmother can tell what the problem is. Most quackery, then, employs healing techniques and products that appear to be similar to those of conventional physicians: drugs, foods, devices, and surgery.[4]

By far the most common form of quack medicine involves drugs, or "medicines," that may be ingested, applied to the skin, or injected. The quack will dispense almost anything that will fit into a bottle, with a sales pitch telling how the wonderful substance will relieve or cure "anything that ails you."

One of the more remarkable chapters of the quack nostrum

3. John Camp, *The Healer's Art*, p. 91.

4. Much of the early work of the Food and Drug Administration and the Federal Trade Commission involved erecting legal barriers to the practices of quacks.

saga featured Harry M. Hoxsey, whose "cancer cures" were known to a generation of Americans and used by thousands.[5] Hoxsey, whose parents both died of cancer, credited his great-grandfather with extracting a cancer cure from an Illinois farm on which a Percheron stallion allegedly was cured of cancer of the right hock by standing knee-deep in a clump of shrubs and flowering plants. The cure, extracted from the shrubs, was presumably passed through the generations to Hoxsey, who first used the secret remedy on a Civil War veteran who claimed to have cancer of the lip, and who thereafter provided endless testimonials to his cure. For surface cancers Hoxsey used a paste, the key ingredient of which was later found to be arsenic, a corrosive chemical that eats away flesh. For internal cancers Hoxsey concocted a secret tonic, later revealed in court actions to consist of potassium iodide, cascara sagrada (an herbal laxative), sugar syrup, prickly ash, buckthorn, alfalfa, red clover blossoms, and pepsin. For this treatment, in 1936, Hoxsey collected three hundred dollars, and over the next twenty years hundreds of thousands of people received his so-called cure. It took a decade of litigation before the Hoxsey treatment was finally stopped in 1960, but the story is noteworthy for the widespread commercial success of the Hoxsey venture and the documentation of ardent belief in it and hostility toward the federal government's attempts to unmask it.

One of the most fertile fields for the quack is food therapy. Until the early part of this century there was very little understanding of the importance of nutrition and diet in maintaining health. With the discovery of specific food and vitamin deficiencies, and the increased public mindfulness of nutrition, quacks quickly began operating on the fringes of legitimacy. Although the new awareness of nutrition was extremely important in providing better health for whole populations, exploitation of the movement was enhanced and abetted by dissemination of the myth of nutritional deficiency as the cause of *most*

5. Young, *The Medical Messiahs*, pp. 360-89.

diseases. According to the basic myth, most diseases can be corrected by proper diet, and by the 1930s in America quacks were having a field day in peddling all sorts of remedies and foods allegedly capable of restoring the body to health and making people capable of extraordinary physical feats. Quacks took advantage of the public's concern for nutrition by concocting worthless potions or foods and selling them as "cures" that could restore hair, build busts, and prevent diseases not present.[6] The nutrition quack uses half-truths, first convincing the prospective buyer of the presence of a nutritional deficiency, then selling foods that are unnecessary and would be unable to avert the danger even if it were present.

Although drug and food quackery are more common, quackery utilizing devices is usually more elaborate and ingenious. This technique of fake healing currently seems to be on the wane, no doubt because present medical devices are so complex and expensive that imitation of them is beyond the individual entrepreneur. In its day, though, device quackery duped the public with machines and gadgets that were supposed to heal by taking bad electricity out of the body, or putting good electricity into the body. One of these was the magnetic or "voltaic" belt, widely distributed toward the end of the nineteenth century. The "Radio Therapeutic Instrument,"[7] used to treat cancer and other maladies, was a machine with many impressive switches and dials to which electrodes were connected, then placed on parts of the body. For each possible diagnosis, which was ascertained through use of the instrument, there was a different setting of the dials. Most quack devices of the day utilized some form of magnetism or electricity, paralleling the popular scientific interests. Some of these devices had nothing inside, or had wires and components incapable of functioning. The widespread use of device quackery pointed to the forthcoming influence of technology in therapeutics. Unquestionably, people were very

6. Ibid., pp. 333-59.
7. Ibid., p. 239.

much impressed by these quack devices, and thousands of patients were convinced that they were "cured" by them. The history of device quackery demonstrates an unequivocal positive effect on patients unrelated to the true benefit of the devices. We would do well to remember this when we consider the triumphs of modern medical technology.

Although quackery commonly is associated only with food, drugs or devices, any health claim that is deliberately untrue or misleading qualifies as quackery, including fraudulent surgery. We might say that the medieval medicine man who hid a piece of bone or metal in his mouth and pretended to suck it out of the patient's body deliberately deceived people and therefore ought to be regarded as a quack. However, whether a practice is considered quackery depends on whether it is sanctioned by the society in which it occurs. There can be no such exemption for modern psychic surgeons who, by magicians' sleight-of-hand tricks, beguile patients into thinking that they have removed or repaired diseased internal organs.[8] Although it is far easier for the average person to attribute healing properties to a drug or mysterious device than it is to believe that someone has operated on him without producing pain or even a scar, the thousands of persons who undergo this experience every year bear witness to belief in this form of healing.

One patient had for twenty years suffered from compression of his heart by a constricting band of calcium (constrictive pericarditis), which caused too much fluid to collect in his body and limited his capacity for exercise. During the early stages of his illness he had two conventional operations to cut away the band of calcium, but both operations failed. After years of disability this unfortunate man made a pilgrimage at considerable expense to a far-off country. There he had "psychic surgery," during which he believes that the calcium around his heart was removed. His positive response to the treatment was beyond question, but X rays of his heart showed all the calcium still in place.

8. George W. Meek, *Healers and the Healing Process*, pp. 107-10, 125.

In objective tests it was found that his heart worked no better and he was not able to do more physically, although he claimed to be tremendously improved by the "operation," and it was apparent that he did *feel* better.

He had been tricked into believing he had had surgery, and had been lied to about removal of the calcium, but he believed in the effectiveness of the treatment, and in his mind he truly experienced healing. This example should make anyone cautious about crediting any sort of operation with a cure without substantial evidence. The word of the patient is not enough. This form of "surgery" is willfully deceptive and misrepresentative, and therefore is quackery.

TECHNIQUES OF QUACKERY

> To advertise any remedy or operation, you have only to pick out all the most reassuring advances made by civilization, and boldly present the two in the relation of cause and effect: the public will swallow the fallacy without a wry face.
>
> George Bernard Shaw,
> *The Doctor's Dilemma*

Post hoc, ergo propter hoc ("after this, therefore because of this") is the great source of the quack's credibility just as it was of the credibility of the first physicians. As the public is always only too eager to associate recovery from sickness with a remedy, the illusion that his remedy is responsible for the cure is easy for the quack to create. This fallacy permeates virtually all aspects of therapeutics, and it is the exceptional person who can avoid it altogether.

The *post hoc, ergo propter hoc* mistake is especially easy to make when the association between "cure" and remedy is made by a doctorlike figure. The successful quack copies traditional medical practices. The patient may realize that the quack is not a legitimate physician, but if the quack can imitate the speech, techniques, promises and authoritativeness of the real physician, it is nearly impossible for the average person to avoid unconsciously associating him with a real doctor.

The mass media practice this technique in advertising. If cough medicine, or vitamins, or even cigarettes are recommended by an actor or model who looks like a physician, the product will sell, not because of its benefit, but because of its association with the image of the physician. The fraudulently assumed authority of quacks should convince anyone of the danger of blindly relying on an authority figure in health matters, and the reader should remember that this is a technique of quackery when we later examine the assumed authority of physicians.

A second basic technique quacks use is suggesting the presence of disease. Obviously, before a person will buy a quack remedy, he must first believe he has the disease the remedy is said to cure. This is why the quack almost always begins by discussing one or more diseases, to plant the fear of illness in the patient. This is actually an easy task for a smooth talker, as everyone has minor aches and discomforts that can be construed as the signs of early disease, given the appropriate and imaginatively portrayed suggestion. A particularly insidious variation of this is the suggestion that a person has a so-called subclinical disease, not detectable either by patient or healer, but nevertheless requiring treatment lest it get out of hand. This specious reasoning finds ready acceptance among all groups. Quacks can convince people to buy remedies to "prevent" cancer, to avoid nutritional deficiencies, or to stop all sorts of diseases before they begin. This ability to get people to treat nonexistent diseases is a far greater tribute to the quack's ingenuity than selling another remedy for arthritis.

A third technique of quackery is persuading people to do what they want to do. The quack knows that almost every person has his own ideas about how to take care of himself. Frequently these ideas disagree with conventional theory, but the individual is usually constrained by conventional medical practice and discouraged by family and associates from unconventional behavior in health matters. The quack encourages personal inclinations by exhorting the patient to "think for yourself." By urging deviance from conventional methods he releases the patient from established patterns of health care and frees him to use the therapy that the quack just happens to have for sale. Once the patient is persuaded to follow his own instincts, always an appealing course of action, he is easy prey for the therapy he associates with his new-found freedom. In the ever-recurring choice between following orthodox therapy, with its known limitations, and opting for a new treatment equally rational to the patient, it is surprising that quack theories do not win out more often.

Of all the ways of imitating established medical practitioners, simulating scientific methods is the quack's most prominent stock in trade. Since scientific advances have given medicine its most dramatic cures, the public associates these triumphs with science and technology. The quack therefore adopts the jargon, the gadgetry and all the trappings of the scientific endeavor. In fact, the quack frequently presents himself as "the scientist ahead of his time," who has made a breakthrough equivalent to the discovery of penicillin. References in the media and by physicians to the "miracles of science" attune the public to the probability of more miracles through scientific advances, a setting virtually demanding quack exploitation of a citizenry that has no understanding of the rigors of science. The glamor of science is distorted to the advantage of the quack, with science and pseudoscience advancing hand-in-hand. The latest quack cancer cure can come from the laboratory, wrapped in computer printouts, as easily as anything sanctioned by the American Cancer Society. When the quack simulates the scientific setting, he is in fact reproducing an important part of the therapeutic setting of modern medicine, and perhaps displaying more insight into the importance of the setting than is acknowledged by conventional physicians.

As quackery operates on the margins of orthodox medicine, it naturally has appeal to persons who can not be helped by conventional medicine. Patients with chronic diseases, such as rheumatoid arthritis or multiple sclerosis, soon learn the limitations of medicine and seek elsewhere for the elusive cure. Similarly, patients who are medical "failures," or those with incurable diseases such as cancer, are particularly prone to the promises of the quack. The "what-have-you-got-to-lose?" sentiment induces many patients to take what seems to be a long-shot gamble, backed by the dubious notion that nothing is lost even if the treatment does not succeed. Find a desperately ill person and you have found someone who is willing to pay any price for the hope of beating the odds. The quack peddles hope.

He could not prosper, however, without the support of the public. The quack obtains public approval through his most reliable technique, the testimonial, without which he could not survive. Quackery capitalizes on the most durable phenomenon in the history of medicine: For any given therapy, no matter how noxious or worthless, there always will be individuals who believe in its benefit. Given that modern placebos consistently have a thirty-five percent success rate, it is no problem to find people willing to testify to the healing power of almost any nostrum. The quack elicits testimonials from a crowd by appealing to the cured to "help your fellow man."

The incredible influence of testimonials on the average person is even stronger when they are written in newspapers and magazines, even though they are as often as not written by the quack himself. Smoothly working quacks will supply an endless outpouring of testimonials, some of them from persons who have had neither the disease nor the therapy. Although the testimonial provides no evidence whatsoever as to the *specific* effect of a therapy, it is almost universally accepted as proof of cure. Thus there is no need, in the minds of the public, for scientific analysis, which in virtually all instances would contradict the testimonials.

IDENTIFYING QUACKERY

If quackery misrepresents by imitating reputable physicians and techniques, how can it be identified as fraudulent by the public?

The quack healer does not allow scrutiny of his methods, and he does not check the results of the therapy. He never assesses with the patient the effect of the treatment, so as to make modifications if necessary. The healer who truly desires to help his patients must above all find out whether he has done so. As a minimum requirement, the therapist should give the patient the opportunity to return so that they can discuss and evaluate the therapy. But the itinerant quack always tries to leave town before there is time for his patients and the public to observe the long-range results of his work. Quacks are particularly fortunate when patients travel long distances to see them, and then return home, making follow-up impossible.

Another feature of quackery is promotional stunts. There are, in fact, very few real cures around, and those are well known and available to the public. Sensationalist advertising by the quack is one reason most members of the medical profession have an aversion to advertising in any form. The quack copies gimmicks used by reputable firms to sell soaps, toothpaste, cigarettes and new cars — meretricious appeals to human instincts and desires. When automobile advertising is filled with half-truths and false claims, readily believed by the public and unquestionably acceptable to society, why shouldn't the quack use the same methods?

Excessive claims are basic in quackery. The truth is, however, that when a remedy is touted as being able to combat a large number of diseases, it very likely is ineffective for all. Really curative medicines not only are few, but they tend to be specific. A particular antibiotic is not effective against all infections, but only against a specific few. A drug that helps to prevent peptic ulcers is of no value in the treatment of kidney disease, and so on. Most quacks can not resist the temptation to claim that their potions will cure almost all diseases, because they usually have only one or two remedies, and to restrict them to one or two diseases would severely limit business. There never has been a universal cure, and any therapy claimed to be effective against "the common cold, wounds, burns, injuries, infections, rheumatic disease, allergies, back trouble, cancer, and the aging process" is virtually always effective against none of them.

A time-honored claim of quacks is that they have a "secret" remedy, not available from other sources. This appeals to people with a certain mentality and insulates the product from competition. Any claim of "miracle" cures is a sure sign of quackery.

The goal of the quack is to exchange deceit for money. Occasionally he may give away a bottle of snake oil as an investment, but quackery is at heart always a commercial enterprise.

REASONS FOR THE SUCCESS OF QUACKERY

It is commonly said that quackery is "the offspring of ignorance." It ought to follow that enlightenment would assure the decline of quackery, but events of the last half century prove otherwise. In spite of substantial governmental and private efforts in recent decades to educate the public to the tricks of quackery, the practice flourishes as much as ever.

Consider Hadacol, which became a national craze in America in 1950. How, in this scientific age, when people are healthier than ever, could the public spend millions of dollars on an elixir consisting of alcohol, B vitamins, iron, calcium, phosphorus, hydrochloric acid and honey?[9] What is so compelling about quackery that it causes educated people to take leave of their reason?

Sociologists and psychologists talk of an innate susceptibility to quackery which can not be eradicated from the human spirit. They say there are deep forces in human nature to which the quack appeals. Clearly, intelligence and education do not protect against quackery. Indeed, there are few among us who never

9. Young, *The Medical Messiahs*, pp. 316-33.

have been taken in by the slick sales pitch, even though common sense ought to have dictated otherwise. When an emotionally desirable belief presents itself, we suspend the critical faculties that usually protect us, however irrational that belief. People who could never be tricked into buying a fake jewel, or who would insist on the most rigorous scrutiny before buying a piece of art or a professional service, sometimes act totally irrationally in matters of health, reverting to what amounts to belief in magic and the occult.

Quackery heals by the same mechanisms that the physicians of antiquity used. The quack gives reassurance, hope and faith in large doses to counteract fear, desperation and anxiety and give the healing force of nature a chance to do its work. And the quack knows how to persuade the patient to associate improvement with the cure, but attribute failure to another cause.

Quack "cures" are sometimes sustained for years. People feel better after quack treatment because of the placebo effect — because they have received healing. But there is more to quackery than preying on the credulity of sick persons. Quackery exists because people want healing and have been conditioned to seek it without differentiating between healing and curing.

In short, the quack capitalizes on the same natural phenomena that have sustained the medical profession from its beginning. The lessons we can learn from quackery are how the mechanisms of its success operate in conventional medicine. So long as patients and physicians can not tell the difference between curative therapies and remedies that enhance nonspecific healing, quackery will always exist.

HEALERS

> And they who first referred this disease to the gods, appear to me to have been just such persons as the conjurors, purifactors, mountebanks, and charlatans now are, who give themselves out for being excessively religious, and as knowing more than other people.
>
> Hippocrates

Although physicians reign supreme in Western societies to-day, healers were dominant in prehistoric times, and one group (homeopaths) actually outnumbered physicians in North America for a time during the nineteenth century. Healers predominate today in many non-Western societies; and even in the modern technological countries, they are popular and influential in health matters.

The theoretical systems of healers and physicians are fundamentally different. Physicians examine diseased tissue and do physiologic and pharmacologic testing. Healers reject these methods. The physician seeks a biological reason for each specific disease and treats it mechanically. The healer works from a general theory which applies to all diseases and therapies and supersedes any particular practice. Fundamentally, the healer aims for healing, which is accomplished through the mind, while the physician aims for curing, which involves manipulation of physical matter.

The healer, therefore, offers the patient a life philosophy to deal with all human problems, not just disease. The philosophy is usually held to be more important than any therapy, and sometimes, as with faith healers, healing may be secondary to spiritual instruction. Healers may use physical methods, such as acupuncture, but the therapeutic effect is attributed to some kind of healing power higher than the physical. Most healers are vitalists—they believe that the healing power comes from an external supernatural force. The various schools, however, do not have identical beliefs: The spiritualist's bioplasmic healing is nonsense to the Christian faith healer, whose religious symbolism is nonsense to the acupuncturist. Other healers—let us call them naturalists—rely not on supernatural forces but on remedies found in nature, such as herbs, the therapeutic powers of which are accepted without reliance on anatomic or physiologic testing, but on empirical evidence or belief.

FAITH HEALERS

The faith healer operates within a belief system in which healing is only one aspect of an encompassing belief in God, usually with strong Christian overtones. Healing comes straight from God through the healer, without drugs, devices or surgery. The lineage of Christian faith healing can be traced back to the shamans, the ancient priest-physicians, and the alchemists. Faith healing can awaken in people their deepest feelings of purpose, being, and relationship to the universe. In the religious person it evokes the ultimate expression of life, disease and death, so that for a true believer, the faith healer is much better able to produce the emotional state of mind conducive to healing than any physician.

Faith healing sometimes is achieved by the "laying on of hands" of the healer, but more commonly the sufferer is healed through oratory or a ceremony. The extent and vitality of faith healing in modern America is visible on national and local television, which faith healers have utilized with enormous success. The key ingredients are the charisma and reputation of the healer, emotional preparation, and the desire of the assembled to see healing. The usual sequence follows that of pretelevision tent meetings. First the religious setting is established with hymns, readings and a sermon. Then the ill are brought forth, the cure is given or pronounced, and the "cured" testify to their healing. The cure is usually attributed to a direct act of God, or Christ, but the healer must induce in the sufferer sufficient faith to receive healing. The healer does this by persuading the individual that the power of God is focused directly upon him.

In television or tent, faith healing alleviates illness but may or may not affect actual diseases. Perhaps the greatest mistake people make about faith healing is to confuse transient relief of symptoms, or improved function (which any inspirational speaker can induce), with lasting improvement or alleviation of suffering, which almost no faith healer is ever around to assess. If the patient improves even for two minutes, the healer is credited, but who checks the patient a week later, or a month later, to see if the improvement has lasted?

The faith healer takes advantage of a universal finding: Almost anyone with a chronic illness can improve his daily functioning if properly motivated. This is because patients with chronic diseases, such as arthritis, polio or heart disease, never function at full capacity on a daily basis. To do so would require giving up being waited upon by others and expending much more effort or enduring much more pain than is worthwhile to the chronic invalid. There is seldom a lame person who can not walk or move somewhat better than he usually does; when the faith healer persuades an invalid to put down his crutches and take a few wobbly steps, which he has not done for years, it is not a miracle, but merely success in inspiring the patient to maximal effort by intense emotional encouragement.

The ability to induce increased function in chronically ill patients and the transient nature of such efforts are described by Benjamin Franklin in the following account:

> Some years since, when newspapers made mention of great cures performed in Italy or Germany, by means of electricity, a number of paralytics were brought to me from different parts of Pennsylvania and the neighboring provinces to be electricised; which I did for them at their request. My method was to place the patient first in a chair, on an electric stool, and draw a number of large strong sparks from all parts of the affected limb or side. Then I fully charged two six-gallon glass jars, each of which had about three square feet of surface coated; and I sent the united shock of these thro the affected limb or limbs; repeating the stroke commonly three times each day. The first thing observed was an immediate greater sensible warmth in the lame limbs that had received the stroke, than in the others; and the next morning the patients usually related that they had in the night felt a pricking sensation in the flesh of the paralytic limbs, and would sometimes shew a number of small red spots, which they supposed were occasioned by those prickings. The limbs too were found more capable of voluntary motion, and seemed to receive strength. A man, for instance, who could not the first day lift the lame hand

from off his knee, would the next day raise it four or five inches, the third day higher; and on the fifth day was able, but with a feeble languid motion, to take off his hat.

These appearances gave great spirits to the patients, and made them hope a perfect cure; but I do not remember, that I saw any amendment after the fifth day; which the patients perceiving, and finding the shocks pretty severe, they became discouraged, went home, and in a short time relapsed; so that I never knew any advantage from electricity in palsies, that was permanent. And how far the apparent temporary advantage might arise from the exercise in the patients' journey, and coming daily to my house, or from the spirits given by the hope of success, enabling them to exert more strength in moving their limbs, I will not pretend to say.[10]

Franklin, in fact, achieved healing through the fifth day of treatment. Had he stopped after the first treatment or the first few, he could have claimed tremendous success and undoubtedly would have been believed. But since he wanted to be sure of the specific effect of the treatment, he persisted and watched his patients relapse after the healing effect had worn off. This is a well-documented observation of the difference between healing and curing, and it shows that Franklin understood the effect of the therapeutic milieu upon healing.

Sometimes it is unclear whether persons who are "cured" actually have the disease in the first place. The modern television healer, for instance, suggests to the audience that persons are present with certain diseases and then, without identifying the people he means, announces the cure. On one television show a healthy-looking young man came up to the stage and told the healer of a lung problem he had had for the past two weeks but had been unaware of until the healer had pointed in his direction five minutes before, saying, "Someone up there has had a lung problem for the last two weeks." The young man related how he at that moment first realized he had the lung

10. Benjamin Franklin, "Account of Effects of Electricity in Paralytic Cases: Letter to J. Pringle, M.D., Jan. 12, 1758," *Philosophical Transcripts* 50(1759):481.

problem and was cured of it in the same instant. The healer replied, "Incipient bronchial emphysema—cured by the Lord." Many illnesses from which people reputedly are cured exist only in the minds of the healer and the persons desiring healing.

At Lourdes and similar shrines the holy place and religious rituals are the intermediaries between the sufferer and God. The process evokes faith, hope, and expectation, the great healing emotions. The total experience of Lourdes, beginning with the idea of going there, is strikingly similar to that of the patients who went to the Aesculapian temples, where the preparation was probably more therapeutic than the final healing ceremony. To the faithful, Lourdes has been a repository of healing power for as long as they have believed. The occasional doubt aside, the lifelong teachings of church, family and culture have suggested in the most potent manner that cures occur at Lourdes. The very act of deciding to go there produces therapeutic hope and expectation.

Most pilgrims to Lourdes have become resigned to chronic diseases resistant to conventional cures. During the period of preparation there is a dramatic change from despair to hope. Friends and family, instead of reflecting hopelessness as in the past, are now the picture of encouragement. Much as the expectation of a vacation can produce a remarkable change in the average worker, preparation for the pilgrimage raises the spirits of the ill person. The travel plans and arrangements for someone to take care of the home while the patient is away marshal the support of the entire community. The attention of family and friends, prayers and special masses, and the salutations and good wishes of all who come into contact with the invalid add to the atmosphere of hope and faith in the holy mission. As the Aesculapian priests well knew, the therapeutic surroundings are the key element, and many a patient is convinced of a sure cure well before arriving at Lourdes.

The time at Lourdes is filled with religious services and trips to the Grotto. Everywhere there are people who have come to witness the miracles. The atmosphere is filled with love, everyone praying for everyone else, the well for the sick, the sick for the other sick. The invalid feels more emotional support than the average person receives in a lifetime, and is surrounded by stories of cures and piles of discarded crutches. The climax is a march to the shrine with hymns, the procession of the priests and the Children of Mary, and fervent prayers, culminating in the raising of the Sacred Host above each sick person.[11]

The intensity and depth of the experience produces an optimal healing atmosphere in which crutches are discarded, the dumb talk, and pain disappears. It is difficult to imagine greater mobilization of the emotional healing forces for those who believe. Although the great majority of patients are not cured, and the population living in the vicinity of Lourdes does not have an increased cure rate, many pilgrims experience profound and dramatic healing.

The phenomenon of Lourdes is an example of the unquestioned therapeutic effect of faith healing, which has elements in common with all other types of healing. The lesson of Lourdes is to be found not in specific cures or claims of miracles, for the experience does not produce *lasting* cures over and above those occurring naturally or through other processes. The greater meaning of Lourdes is the immense and real response of ill persons to the therapeutic setting of hope, belief and love.

Faith healing produces dramatic and, at times, real benefit for those who are healed. My intention is not to deride or decry it, or any type of healing, but to examine its mechanisms and limitations, and, in a later chapter, its place in modern medical practices.

ACUPUNCTURE

Many Westerners think that acupuncture is used predominantly for anesthesia, but in fact the Chinese did not use it in

---

11. Jerome D. Frank, *Persuasion and Healing*, pp. 67-72.

surgery until 1958, although it is almost five thousand years old. It is mentioned in the oldest Chinese book on medicine, and is practiced not only for alleviation of pain, but for treatment of disease. It is performed by inserting very fine needles into the body at specific points called loci, through which energy is supposed to flow and restore balance to the organs and the whole person. In the Chinese culture, acupuncture is a philosophy of life, of which healing is only one part.

According to this belief, the forces behind life and death manifest themselves in Ch'i, the equivalent of vital energy. The flow of Ch'i through the body is controlled by the interplay of two opposing forces, the yin and the yang, the yin being negative and the yang positive. Health results from a balance of the forces of yin and yang, while disease represents an imbalance of these forces. The acupuncturist practices preventive medicine, but if an imbalance is discovered by the appearance of symptoms, treatment is possible at that stage as well.

Acupuncture is intriguing to Westerners because it defies our conceptions of physiology. To the average Westerner open-heart surgery under acupuncture anesthesia is incomprehensible, and that the chest could be opened without collapse of the lungs seems equally inexplicable. The Westerner can only attempt to explain acupuncture anesthesia through biological concepts, such as a "spinal-gate" theory of pain interruption. Such analysis, however, misses the mark, for acupuncture is not posited on a physical system. Physical instruments and techniques are used, but the purpose is to adjust the flow of the vital force, an unmeasurable entity. For the user, the balance of yin and yang explains everything in creation: heaven, earth, life and disease. In the flow of vital energy through the acupuncture needles the patient perceives a balance or harmony without which a cure is held to be impossible.

Acupuncture does not cure diseases such as cancer, heart disease or trauma, but for those who accept its premises, it is as potent a healing force as faith is for the Christian, and healing is difficult or impossible without it. It induces the feeling of completeness, oneness or rightness with the world from which the feeling of wellness flows. A Westerner who thinks acupuncture is akin to witchcraft can not derive benefit from it because it does not evoke for him the necessary healing responses.

NATURALISTS

The belief system of chiropractic was formulated by "DD" Palmer, who previously had practiced phrenology and mesmerism, which he discarded in favor of the new "science" of adjusting spines so as to "relieve any impingement on the delicate nerve fibers." According to the chiropractic principle, the innate life-giving force of nature flows down the spinal canal, and any impingement on the canal results in disease. Palmer's new system of anatomy consisted of four circulatory systems (reminiscent of the Galenic humors), and he related all human illnesses to subluxations of the spine.[12] The chiropractic belief system may not be congruous with modern biophysical principles, but at the turn of the last century when chiropractic was taking hold, and even today, it was as believable to many people as the complex theories advanced by physicians.

Chiropractic does not claim supernatural powers, but relies on "natural healing." The widespread popularity of chiropractic and its persistence as an alternative to conventional medicine are due in no small part to the appeal of healing through "natural" means—in this case manipulations—rather than "unnatural" drugs and operations (although the chiropractor does simulate science with gadgets and extensive use of X rays of the spine).

The chiropractor believes that by adjusting bones he adjusts

12. J.M. Luce, "Chiropractic—Its History and Challenge to Medicine," *Pharos* 41(1978):12; George S. Mills, *Rogues and Heroes from Iowa's Amazing Past*, p. 234; D.V. McQueen, "The History of Science and Medicine as Theoretical Sources for the Comparative Study of Contemporary Medical Systems," *Social Science and Medicine* 12(1978):69; G. Dunea, "Healing by Touching," *British Medical Journal* 1(1979):795.

muscles, which in turn adjust organs, the process leading to a reorganization of the whole body and the social and psychological life of the patient. The person who is able to feel and hear his neck move and can associate the act with feeling better often finds both the explanation of disease and the source of healing more consistent with his overall life-philosophy than the obfuscation and dependency he finds in orthodox medical care.

Chiropractic serves many patients and is a major alternative to conventional medicine. It survives not because of the accuracy of its claims, which are largely unmeasurable and not scientifically validated, but because of its ability to heal. This success is epitomized by the stock-in-trade of the chiropractor, treatment of low back pain. This malady, perhaps the most ubiquitous in the human species, is the archetypical chronic disease, with bothersome recurrences followed by natural remissions, allowing no permanent cure. It is poorly treated by conventional physicians, but susceptible to natural recovery.

By depending primarily on testimonials for confirmation, and by treating only chronic or self-limited disorders, the chiropractor has gained acceptance as a healer who takes the time to talk to his patient, always gives an understandable explanation of illness, and always promises a cure. The combination of simulated science, palatable belief system, and willingness to attend to the basic emotional needs of patients is enough to bring success to this group of healers.

In like manner, naturopaths, herbalists, and others advocate a holistic philosophy of natural healing which mixes pseudoscience, herbs, manipulation, psychic therapy and almost all forms of treatment that satisfy nonspecific therapeutic requirements. These healers succeed by giving believable explanations of disease, using treatments that seem "natural" and therefore mesh with their patients' values and beliefs, and practicing the nonspecific methods of healing. In common with other unconventional healers, they have no systematic or scientific means of assessing specific effects or benefit of their therapies.

PSYCHIC HEALERS

A modern variation of belief in the supernatural cause of
health and disease is expressed in concepts of "higher-
consciousness" or "other-consciousness" energies or forces. A
psychic healing force is but one part of an encompassing life-
philosophy which explains and directs all existences in the
cosmos. Terms used to describe interaction between psychic
forces and human consciousness are *astral travel, bioplasmic* or
etheric bodies, antimatter, negative space-time and *out-of-body
experience.* In simple terms, psychics believe in a supernatural
force capable of interacting with all organisms. It is unmeasurable by material standards and undescribable by usual language.
It communicates by electromagnetism, vibrations or other
mechanisms largely incomprehensible to the conscious human
mind. There are numerous permutations of the basic belief in a
spirit force, some admixed with established religions and others
not, the latter group being in conflict with organized religions.

Healing is achieved by the individual patient or through a
healer. Self-healing begins by attaining a "higher" self, which is
done by passing through a stage of *wanting* to become healthy
and into a stage of meditation, "attunement" or "at-one-ment"
leading to "knowing," the state of optimal health in which the
patient "knows" he is healthy. Visualizing oneself as "whole,
healthy, vibrant, free of disease" is an important technique, the
endpoint being a feeling akin to the ecstasy of writers, a sense of
abiding peace, a oneness with nature, and a total engagement
with the emotions of "love, compassion, equanimity, quietness,
and confidence."[13] The pathway to individual health, then, is
the same for the psychic as for the mystic or the Christian or the
Oriental who strives for nirvana. It is the realization of the
healing emotional state.

Psychic healing administered by a practitioner, however, is a
more complex affair in which the healer uses presumed powers

13. Meek, *Healers and the Healing Process,* p. 176.

to "cure" the patient, who is relatively passive. The best known of these healers, the psychic surgeons of the Philippines, are remarkable for their claims of healing by bloodless surgery in which they "enter" the body and "remove" or rearrange diseased organs without leaving a physical trace of having done so. This is a modification of the usual form of psychic healing in that actual physical changes are claimed. Success of the technique is supported by thousands who have given testimony to its healing effect. The healers most assuredly employ sleight-of-hand techniques to produce an illusion of surgery,[14] in a manner similar to shamans who pretended to extract tissues, but the important point about psychic healing is not whether the techniques constitute dupery. Most emphatically, the lesson in the context of modern medicine is that both healer and patient believe in the power of the healer and in the accomplishments he claims. In the objective, scientific, materialistic sense psychic surgery is a sham, but in the symbolic sense it is real and results in healing.

PSYCHOTHERAPISTS

Although psychiatrists are, by our definition, physicians because they hold the M.D. degree, in many ways they and other psychotherapists are more like healers than physicians, for they work with the unmeasurable functions of the mind and achieve, for the most part, healing instead of curing. In Western medicine, which treats mind and body as separate entities, psychotherapists are the link between body-oriented physicians and mind-oriented healers. Freud's greatest contribution may be viewed as linking the physical world of illness with the mental world through the unconscious mind rather than the supernatural.

Although psychiatrists are retreating more and more from psychodynamic interpretations of diseases such as schizophre-

14. Richard Grossinger, *Planet Medicine*, p. 191.

nia, toward biochemical interpretations, they have for the most part treated emotional disorders with a variety of specific techniques all aimed at producing the same nonspecific healing environment. Whether a psychotherapist approaches an emotional disorder through conventional psychoanalysis, insight therapy, behaviorism, screaming, immersion in warm water, or unmitigated verbal abuse, the goal of the therapy, nonspecific healing, is the same. In other words, although a patient may be helped by one specific psychotherapeutic technique more than by another, the various techniques have elements in common: encouragement, rational explanation of the problem, reason for hope, support, positive experiences, help in reliving the origin of distress, and reassurances that produce a tranquil emotional state.

The goal of psychotherapy when applied to physical disorders is clearly to induce in the patient an emotional state supportive of natural healing, a sense of healthiness, a wish to be healed, and in general a positive outlook. In its goals, effects and successes it is no different from psychic healing, faith healing or the healing ceremonies of the Navaho Indians, except that it is couched in terms consistent with the Western belief system.

Characteristics of Healers

What do all these different kinds of healers have in common? First, they all rely upon nonspecific means of healing, and do not achieve curing directly. They use unmeasurable healing forces—supernatural or allegedly natural—and do not assess results by any scientific means. Like the early physicians they take credit for natural healing and disclaim responsibility for failures. Clinical records of before-and-after states are not kept by faith healers and psychic healers, and there is no way of knowing whether the diseases patients are treated for actually existed either before or after therapy. Cures are declared by the healer and supported solely by testimonials of the healed. The faith healer brushes aside failure by claiming "the patient did not want to be healed," or "God did not intend this patient to get well." Psychics explain failures by the absence of sufficient desire of the patient to get well, and homeopaths deny some treatment failures by explaining the diseases as "necessary for survival of the patient," or as "protecting the mental plane."[15]

Healers take advantage of the transient effects of healing. Like the quack, intention notwithstanding, the healer does not check on the long-term results of his ministrations. What happens to the person with cancer, who in reacting to the emotional intensity of the faith healer gives testimony of being healed? All studies of the subject show that such persons die at the same alarming rate as other persons with cancer. When the experience of Lourdes wears off after the return home, who tells the world that the invalid can walk no better than before the visit? In not assessing the long-term effects of therapy, the healer is quintessentially unscientific and not different from the quack.

A characteristic common to many healers is the rationalization of deceptive techniques in the name of helping patients. The ends justify the means, and the patient's testimony to well-being is held as sufficient cause to use any method in order to "benefit" the patient. Although many healers deny any deceptive tricks in their practices, others acknowledge the use of deception to induce the healing milieu. A psychic surgeon, for instance, can claim that a spirit is guiding his hands during the treatment, so that what would otherwise be sleight-of-hand technique is really only the work of the spirit. One expert on psychic healing points to the deceptive healing effects of placebos physicians use, and to the healing effects of the emotional states produced by acupuncture needles, kneeling in a confessional, reading from the Bible, or reclining on a psychiatrist's couch. He argues that the deception of psychics is no worse than that of other healers, and that final judgment rests on the benefit to the patient. In the words of this advocate:

15. Ibid.

The benefited patient cares nothing about the process — he is just happy to be well again. But with the new insights we have into the nature of illness, healing, and health it behooves us to do everything in our power to enhance the placebo effect.[16]

This is defense of illusion.

When his patients get well, the healer comes to believe not only in his technique but in his innate healing power. This process is well described in a story about how shamans "suck" diseases out of patients, from a book on the religion of the Kwakiutl Indians of Vancouver Island.[17] The story is summarized by Richard Grossinger:

An Indian, who is later to take the shaman name Quesalid, does not believe in the medicine men's ability to cure illness. He thinks they are charlatans and intends to expose this. He hangs out with them until they invite him to join their society. Once inside, he learns that they work by a mixture of practical knowledge, acting, and secrets from paid spies. Most notably, he discovers how when the shaman sucks the disease out of the sick one: he conceals a tuft of down in the corner of his mouth which he vomits up, covered with blood from his biting his tongue, at the height of the healing crisis. This hoax is passed off as the extraction of the disease.

Quesalid is now in a position to expose the entire system, but he decides first to learn more. Before he has a chance to make his public statement, he is trapped by circumstance. A sick person, hearing of his apprenticeship, summons him for help. He "succeeds," at least to the satisfaction of this first client and, thereafter, is known as a great healer and hired to cure many other diseases. Although somewhat disturbed by the turn of events, he holds to his original cynicism and passes off his success as the belief of his patients in him.

Numerous successes undermine his cynicism, and he gains a strange confidence and bravado. He transcends methodology and strides around as a healer-at-large. He has no explanation. But he regards the world differently. He sees his power as something authentic, something he has earned.[18]

16. Meek, *Healers and the Healing Process*, p. 228.
17. Franz Boas, *The Religion of the Kwakiutl Indians*, Part 2: *Translations*, pp. 17-18.
18. Grossinger, *Planet Medicine*, pp. 91-92.

To Quesalid, or any healer, the "extraction" of diseased tissue by a sleight-of-hand technique is allowable because the physical deception is nothing more than an outward expression of the triumph of the healer over the disease. The healer is free of guilt for his deception because he believes that the only important thing is that he has removed the disease from the patient's body. "For the benefit of the patient" is a rationalization physicians as well as healers use to cover a multitude of sins.

CARING AND CURING

While curing depends on biophysical remedies, healing is often primarily the result of caring. A patient who has successful surgery for the removal of a tumor may be cured of disease, but may have a remaining illness due to fear about his condition. Another patient with cancer who goes to a faith healer may respond so dramatically that his illness is eliminated, even though the disease itself remains. Both patients would benefit from a clearer understanding of the difference between curing and healing, for the first needs further caring while the second doesn't grasp the need for curing.

The interrelationships among caring, healing and curing are complex. Healing sometimes accelerates curing, but healing is not the equivalent of curing. The psychic healer may be correct in pointing out the profound influence of the psyche on the body, and in some instances somatic symptoms may be totally abolished by healing alone, but the trouble is that the psyche can not be manipulated in a predictable and consistent manner to produce curing, and transient healing proves to be inadequate in the long run.

There are times when curative treatment is the most effective and efficient means to healing—as in treating pneumonia with penicillin. The patient's life must be saved before his psyche can be soothed. Healing may be approached through caring, curing or an appropriate mix of the two, according to the underlying problem of the patient. It is often the case, however, that healing and curing are distinct functions. Failure to recognize the difference between them frequently puts doctor and patient at cross-purposes.

It is ironical that the ability to cure—an historically recent achievement—makes the modern physician less inclined to caring. If the old-time physician cared for his patients because he had nothing else to do, the modern physician doesn't care for his patients because he has something else to do. Medical students are taught to react to medical problems with curative measures—how to correct diabetic acidosis, how to reconstruct a deformed limb, or how to treat hypertension—but not how to recognize nonphysical sources of distress and the need for caring. Physicians do understand at times that they are giving emotional support, but they confuse attempts to find and cure disease with actual caring for the patient. They respond to almost all pleas for caring by administering curative therapy—a drug or an operation. They are not comfortable with caring because its effects are not measurable; it produces no useful statistics. When asked for evidence of the value of clinical medicine, physicians answer by citing mortality rates and hospital discharges.

Nor do patients understand the difference between curing and caring. In order to gain the physician's attention, they learn to express their feelings in physical terms, such as headache or pain in the chest. The symptoms expressed by the patient may have little to do with the underlying problem, but once the problem is defined in physical terms, the patient gets attention through the drug or the operation. It is the rare patient who leaves the doctor's office without a prescription.

A 49-year-old man was referred to a heart specialist because of chest pain. At the time he was having increasing marital discord because of his inability to fulfill the sexual desires of his wife, who was ten years younger. In an attempt to rationalize his sexual retrenchment, he complained of pain in the chest and fatigue during intercourse. His wife insisted that he see the doctor, to whom he related the problem of chest pain with physical activity. After numerous medical tests, which showed some minor coronary artery disease, the patient submitted to the advice of both his wife and the doctor that he "do something about it," and had coronary bypass surgery. Following the recuperative period, he said he felt well, but was unable to engage in sexual activity, for which his wife left him.

The patient's problem, decline of sexual activity, called for caring and understanding. The physician perceived the problem as a physical one, found a possible physical cause of it, and applied a physical solution.

It is bad enough that patients want or need caring while today's clinicians want to supply curing, but it is much worse that the two don't understand each other's desires. Since neither patients nor physicians differentiate between curing and caring, they tend to interpret the desires of the other as an expression of their own interests. Thus, while the patient misinterprets the doctor's attempts to cure as an expression of caring, the doctor misinterprets the patient's plea for care as a need for curing. In case after case this misunderstanding makes for deficient medical care.

Perhaps it is the lack of caring in physicians that drives people to quacks and healers who can not cure but peddle healing. If caring is all a patient needs, he may be better off with such a healer, but it is a shame that he has to choose between the two. Most of the problems of health care arise from not understanding the proportions of curing and caring a patient needs and how he can best go about getting them.

CHAPTER FOUR

The Doctor-Patient Contract

Physicians should, therefore, minister to the sick with due impressions of the importance of their office; reflecting that the ease, the health, and the lives of those committed to their charge, depend on their skill, attention and fidelity. They should study, also, in their deportment, to unite *tenderness* with *firmness*, and *condescension* with *authority*, as to inspire the minds of their patients with gratitude, respect and confidence.

> American Medical Association
> "Code of Medical Ethics," 1847

Molière saw through the doctors; but he had to call them in just the same. Napoleon had no illusions about them; but he had to die under their treatment just as much as the most credulous ignoramus that ever paid sixpence for a bottle of strong medicine.

> George Bernard Shaw,
> *The Doctor's Dilemma*

THE OMNIPOTENT DOCTOR AND THE HELPLESS PATIENT

SINCE THE first physicians were in effect priests, their cultural descendants have inherited the priestly vestments of aloofness, special powers and access to the supernatural.[1] Historically, the physician has enjoyed prestige, social respect and recently wealth, and has been granted a power to intervene unprecedented in voluntary human relationships. The patient's ignorance of the reasons for his distress, and his belief that only

1. The similarity of modern physicians to the priests from whom they are descended is noted in the writings of critics of modern medicine, who liken hospitals to temples, and medical procedures to religious rites. (Ivan Illich, *Medical Nemesis*, pp. 105-10; Samuel Shem, *The House of God*.)

the physician has the knowledge and power to give relief from distress have made him dependent on the physician and supplicant before him.

This unequal doctor-patient relationship is instilled in the individual in his formative years, probably by the time he is five years old. The relationship of the infant or child patient to the physician is set by the parents and the physician long before the child has any ability to influence it. The awe of the parents for the doctor is transferred to the child.[2] The alacrity with which the doctor's commands are carried out gives them precedence over those of the parents, so that in the child's mind the authority and mysterious power of the doctor supersede the authority of the parents. The physician is the only one who is allowed to violate the rules and taboos of the home, entering the bedroom and physically handling the child's body in an atmosphere in which everything is subordinated to his wishes. The physician is above family law in ordering the mother to get this, or do that, while other household activities cease in deference to his presence.

In the doctor's office and at the hospital, submission to the physician's wishes is even more impressive, with the secretary and nurses who prepare the child for the encounter doing the doctor's bidding. By the time the child grows to the age where he could otherwise enter into a relationship on his own terms, he has learned to accept the power of the doctor to set rules, make pronouncements and give orders, and he has long since come to believe in the doctor's ability to cure. This special ability, coupled with the doctor's routine violation of the usual social and physical taboos, set him apart from other members of society as an extraordinary person whose position and pronouncements should not be challenged. The attitudes toward physicians instilled by both society and family are carried forward throughout life and are very difficult to unfix. Patients who later in life

2. Richard H. Blum, J. Sadusk and R. Waterson, *The Management of the Doctor-Patient Relationship*, p. 68.

challenge either dependency on the physician or the physician's authority are in conflict not only with the doctor but with their previous values and the attitudes of family and friends.

The exalted position of the physician is reinforced in the child's mind through television commercials and "doctor" soap operas, deference given to physicians in public places, the role of physicians in literature and cinema, and the association of physicians with wealth and prestige. Indeed, the title "Dr." sets the physician aside as someone extraordinary, for the child who is taught to call most elders "Mr." or "Mrs." can not escape the distinction of the preferential form of address. In Ecclesiastes we are told to honor the physician because God has created him to serve man's needs. Many children who are taught this retain a life-long association of doctors with religion. At every turn society readies the infant mind for subservience to the physician.

It is self-evident that any child who grows to adulthood has survived all encounters with physicians, and like his forefathers, he has learned to attribute recovery from illness to the ministrations of the physician. A four-year-old may not understand the viral origin of measles or the natural course of the disease, but he does associate getting well with the arrival of the doctor and his medicines. This powerful fixed association strengthens, reinforces and perpetuates the relationship of the helpless child to the powerful healer. In order to receive the benefits of the physician's assumed power, the patient must continue to believe in that power, and therefore must accept a relationship based on an inherent difference between doctor and patient even after he grows up. If one wishes a priest to intercede with God, one must believe that the priest has special access to God. If the physician has no special status, the patient can receive no special healing from him. The adult patient has a deep-seated, long-standing emotional investment in believing.

SURROGATE HEALERS

Since some physicians now practice in partnership, some

patients develop relationships with groups of doctors rather than only one. It is not uncommon for a pregnant woman to discuss the relative merits of her "group," not knowing which physician will preside over the delivery. In the same way, patients who go to large hospitals or clinics tend to develop a relationship with the entire hospital staff, especially if they are likely to see a different physician every visit. The patient who is unable to attribute extraordinary healing power to an individual in an ongoing relationship tends to shift the presumed source of power to the institution, which assumes the role of healer in his mind.[3]

Other patients confer the role of healer on instruments or devices.[4] Patients who are dependent on breathing machines no doubt develop relationships with these machines, and those who are dependent on artificial heart pacemakers often attribute supernatural powers to the devices. It is remarkable how often patients come to believe that the heart can not stop with an artificial pacemaker in place, and that the pacemaker provides additional strength and vitality. The ordinary physician usually can outperform the instrument in the caring role, but if the specific healing function is identified with an instrument, the instrument-patient relationship may take precedence over the doctor-patient relationship.

Not without reason many patients increasingly view advanced technology as the source of healing, but in so doing they transfer to it the same expectation, hope and dependency they feel for the doctor. The endless quest of many patients for a drug, operation or mechanical device promising improved health gives contemporary expression to the age-old act of surrendering to the agent of healing. But it is still the physician who creates and has access to the technology, and the surrender of the

3. S. W. Bloom and P. Summey, "Models of the Doctor-Patient Relationship: A History of the Social System Concept," in The Doctor-Patient Relationship in the Changing Health Scene, ed. Eugene Gallagher, DHEW Publication No. (NIH) 78-183, p. 39.

4. Edgar Berman, The Solid Gold Stethoscope, p. 13.

patient to the physician and his instruments is the main element of the doctor-patient relationship.

THE BASIC CONTRACT

Under the basic unwritten contract, the physician is deeded a special status within society, plus financial compensation, in return for which he uses his special knowledge and power to heal those who are included in the contract. In its simple form a witch doctor or shaman attends to the needs of all members of a community in return for suitable social and material compensation. Modern forms of patient-doctor or patient-group medical relationships are socially and economically more complex, but the terms remain generally the same.

The basic contract holds that the patient must have trust in the doctor.[5] The physician is granted authority to do what he deems necessary, including transgressing personal boundaries, without questioning by the patient.[6] The doctor is given control over the relationship and all acts within it because of his expertise and his benevolent intent. Control by the doctor is a central concept, and under the contract the patient acknowledges the physician's jurisdiction over a wide range of activities in which he must not interfere.[7]

For his part, the doctor agrees to serve the patient, but as even this service is directed and defined by the physician, it is subject to professional standards and the good will of the physician. Ideally, the contract would reflect a reciprocal relationship in which doctor and patient are responsive to each other's needs, but as the doctor is accorded control over all interactions, professional service more closely resembles philanthropy.[8] The physician feels that the contract gives him the "right" to control

5. Marcia Millman, The Unkindest Cut, pp. 179-98.
6. Eliot Freidson, Profession of Medicine, p. 355.
7. Albert R. Jonsen, The Rights of Physicians, p. 8; Judith P. Swazey, Health, Professionals, and the Public, p. 7.
8. Swazey, Health, Professionals, and the Public, p. 10.

all aspects of the relationship, going so far as to construe some obviously nonmedical decisions as medical ones, such as whether the patient should be allowed to die at home or must stay in the hospital.

The individual doctor-patient contract may vary from one of total authority and domination by the physician to one of essentially equal partnership, but the quid pro quo of the contract grants the physician professional authority and autonomy, for which he agrees to take care of the patient.[9]

Sociologists put the doctor-patient relationship into three categories.[10] In the first category the physician is dominant and active, while the patient is inferior, passive and totally dependent. He has blind trust in the physician and never expresses an opinion about management of his problem. The patient is assumed to know nothing, and no attempt is made to include him in decision making. This category includes unconscious patients.

In the next category the physician remains dominant, but the patient is accorded some say in the management of his case. This is probably the most common practice today, although it is similar to an adult-child relationship in which the childlike patient does what the physician says, with few avenues of appeal.

The third category is mutual participation, in which doctor and patient are equal partners in an adult-adult relationship. This sort of relationship is rare because few physicians are willing to share authority on medical decisions, and most patients, whether they realize it or not, want the doctor to take full responsibility for their health. Most mutual participation relationships arise in cases of chronic disease, such as chronic renal failure, where there is a long and intensely personal relationship

9. C.B. Chapman, "On the Definition and Teaching of the Medical Ethic," *New England Journal of Medicine* 301(1979):632.

10. Thomas S. Szasz and M.H. Hollender, "The Basic Models of the Doctor-Patient Relationship," *Archives of Internal Medicine* 97(1956):586.

between doctor and patient, and participation by the patient relieves the physician of the encumbering responsibilities of the patient's daily life. For the patient with a transplanted kidney, mutual participation means the dependent patient has full understanding of a program he must comply with. So long as the physician's authority is not challenged, he is willing to concede lesser decisions and responsibilities.

Central to the contract is the notion of the physician as exclusive healer. The patient may learn from the doctor how to take care of himself, but he may not participate as a healer. This concept is emphasized in the remarks of the editor of a leading medical journal, who fears that consumer education would invade the physician's jurisdiction.

> It is astonishing to hear demands that the patient should be allowed to make major therapeutic decisions. An effective therapeutic relationship requires an atmosphere of trust and confidence and no amount of consumer education can substitute for reliance on the skillful and dedicated guidance of the physician. The need for the preservation of this relationship clearly identifies what consumer education should and should not be . . . .
> We must be alert to the dangers of programs that obscure the distinction between healer and sufferer.[11]

The basic contract recognizes and de facto mandates the therapeutic relationship in which the doctor is granted exclusive power as healer. The public grants exclusive healing privileges to the medical profession through licensing and other means. Virtually all other parts of the contract flow from this concession which is based on the psychological needs of persons to have healers with superhuman characteristics, and which is the fountainhead of the power and success of physicians. The exclusivity, dominance and autonomy of the medical profession derive from and depend on the basic contract, which has been sanctioned by every society.

11. A. Soffer, "Consumer's Rights in Medicine," *Archives of Internal Medicine* 138(1978):905.

THE PHYSICIAN'S CONTROL OVER THE PATIENT

There is nothing worse in the practice of medicine, or anything more destructive and degrading to both patient and physician, than the control the physician exercises over the patient under an unequal contract. The physician demands that the patient give up two fundamental rights, the right to know and the right to decide. These demands are not made orally or in writing—they usually are only partial, and the physician may even be unaware of them—but they are enforced through the tradition of the basic contract.

The physician assumes that his superior knowledge and experience enable him to judge what the patient needs. Since the patient is presumed to be unable to make an informed decision and likely to choose wrongly even if fully informed, it is standard practice for physicians to manipulate information in order to persuade patients to accept recommendations; in fact (as I shall explain in detail in Chapter 5), students are taught by the example of their clinical teachers that such techniques are "in the patient's best interests." Thus the patient is systematically denied the data he needs to make an informed decision. Professional expertise in making medical decisions is indispensable, but withholding pertinent information cheats the patient. In reality, the patient's best interests are served when he, not the doctor, decides what he needs to know. It is hard to imagine that a reasonable patient would want to have important information withheld from him.

Once the physician gains control, he assumes power to make decisions on behalf of the patient, often imposing personal values and ideologies on what are moral and social decisions. Made in the name of "science" and "the good of the patient," medical decisions conform more to the wishes of the physician than those of the patient. Even the traditional position of the woman giving birth, on her back with feet up in stirrups, is for the convenience of the doctor rather than the mother, who would have less pain with greater safety for the baby in a more upright position.[12]

Physicians have so much control that they sometimes usurp the decision of how much pain or disability a patient should tolerate. A 64-year-old man had mild chest pain with exercise, but remained active and was able to hike ten miles in a day. The patient took medicines when necessary and was satisfied with his life style. The physician, however, looked upon the occasional chest pain as an abnormality and recommended a corrective operation. The patient resisted, stating that he was willing to live with his mild disability. But the physician continued to insist until the patient submitted to the operation. Following recovery from the operation, there was no change in the patient's pain.

This was not a case of the physician acting as benevolent parent to help a child who was unable to make a wise decision or to save the patient's life. The patient was fully informed; he understood the potential gains and risks, and was capable of making a decision on the grounds of his own interests. What is important is not the result, which could have been different, but that the physician expropriated the decision about how much pain was tolerable. Physicians control not only the physical aspects of disease, but how patients are allowed to react to them. Thus the physician becomes the enemy by preventing the patient from doing what he wants to do, in the name of the physician's conception of what is right.

How do physicians gain such control over the decisions that rightly belong to the patient? Often by the patient's trust in their judgment; often by reasonable persuasion based on facts; but too often by coercion. Convinced of the rightness of their decisions, physicians will not hesitate to use what they call persuasion, but what is known as coercion in other spheres of life, to gain their ends. They intimidate with threats of a worsening condition or

12. P.M. Dunn, "Obstetric Delivery Today: For Better or for Worse?" *Lancet* 1(1976):790.

death if the patient does not relent to the demand for treatment or diagnostic procedure. The physician's conscious belief in the correctness of the act does not mitigate the patient's resulting loss of control. Resort to intimidation is almost reflexive, and certainly it is professionally acceptable behavior, if the physician is not getting his way. He says things like, "If you don't let us do this test, we won't know what's happening and can't help you," or, "If we don't operate, you'll probably die." Both examples are designed to induce a state of helplessness and dependency in the patient which make him too weak to resist.

This practice is shamelessly, if unconsciously, accepted by physicians and taught as a matter of course to medical students. It is a direct outgrowth of not viewing problems from the patient's perspective, and is rationalized as "knowing what is best and using every means to attain it." Although occasionally questioned by nurses and other nonphysician hospital personnel, it is an integral part of the physician's therapeutic arsenal. The physician knows that he holds the trump card, that in time he can wear the patient down, that rupturing the therapeutic relationship would be devastating to the dependent patient, and that few patients can resist. If resistance is severe, the physician ups the ante, often threatening to sever the relationship. Many a time, just before approaching a patient with a de facto ultimatum, the physician has said to a colleague, "Don't worry, I'll get him; he won't be able to refuse." This is a trick of the quack: creation of distress so that the patient may then be cured.

Control over the patient is nowhere more nearly complete than in the hospital, for here the patient is clearly on the physician's turf, and he must act and respond according to the physician's concept of what is best.[13] Nurses, social workers and orderlies may be sympathetic and offer advice to the patient, but

13. Patients commonly give up basic rights when they enter a hospital. In the introduction to a handbook on the rights of hospital patients, the Director of the Center for Law and Health Science, Boston University School of Law, has written: "The American medical consumer possesses certain interests, many of which may properly be described as rights, that he does not automatically forfeit

from the moment of entry into what many call the temple of medicine, the patient loses control. At the beginning, there is a symbolic exchange of the patient's clothes for depersonalizing hospital garb. The patient is put in a dependent position in bed (often unnecessarily), personal belongings are taken away, family and friends are restricted primarily for the convenience of the hospital staff, and all activities come under the control of the physician and his surrogates. The physician usually does not tell the patient everything that will be done, although major activities — such as examinations or tests requiring insertion of tubes or incisions — and major therapy are usually discussed in advance. The patient learns about everything else when the nurse tells him or the orderly arrives to take him to the designated room or department. Many tests that are considered routine by the hospital staff are anything but routine for the patient. The apparent absence of financial restraints in the hospital has removed the only reason for prior consultation with the patient about activities the physician deems necessary.

There is remarkable inconsideration for the patient's wishes and feelings. Without prior notification, he will be whisked off to a two-hour laboratory test, leaving a friend or relative unable to complete a visit. Many physicians will not think twice about interrupting a patient in the middle of a meal to draw blood or do an examination. Most unfortunate of all is the patient who enters the hospital at night, needing above all rest and sleep. Especially in teaching hospitals this patient is likely to be kept up hours for routine interviews and examinations, all to satisfy professional needs.

Although many patients have learned to expect loss of freedom in the hospital, what they get is humiliating by any other standard. The loss of amenities and the aggravating experience

by entering a hospital; most hospitals fail to recognize the existence of these interests and rights, fail to provide for their protection and assertion, and frequently limit their exercise without recourse for the patient." (George J. Annas, *The Rights of Hospital Patients,* p. 1.)

of lying on a stretcher waiting to be taken to a laboratory test are pardonable inconveniences that may be attributed to poor management, understaffing and the social conditions of institutional life. But the real humiliation, the degradation, is the attitude of the physician and the extent of his control.

Physicians themselves perhaps never experience such humiliation; indeed, they would never stand for it. It is well known that the "worst" patients are doctors and nurses—worst in the sense of not putting up with the dictates of other doctors and nurses. If a physician-as-patient were asked to put on his slippers and go for a barium enema about which he neither was informed nor gave consent, he would not only resolutely refuse to go, but he would register a complaint of sufficient strength that the incident would never be repeated with him. But the ordinary patient puts up with discourtesies and inconveniences that would be intolerable in nonmedical life.

Once in a hospital, the patient's degree of control may be measured by his difficulty in obtaining discharge. He may negotiate his release, but the final decision is the physician's. The same techniques of coercion and intimidation used to gain approval for tests or treatment are used to keep the patient in the hospital. The ultimate intimidation is requiring the patient who insists upon leaving to sign out "against medical advice." In this procedure, the patient must put in writing his intention to disobey the doctor's orders, and acknowledge that by so doing, he may jeopardize his right to future admission to that hospital. Doctors claim the device is used to emphasize the seriousness of the situation to the patient and to protect the doctor from malpractice suits, both claims being legitimate some of the time. However, there are alternative means of accomplishing both of these objectives, such as a clear note on the chart, or even a written statement witnessed and signed by the patient, outlining the physician's reasons for recommending that he stay in the hospital, but without the implication in signing out "against medical advice" that the physician is right and the patient is wrong, an implication an ignorant judge or magistrate might accept. This sign-out requirement is a spurious legitimization of the control of the physician over the patient that strips him of his rights. The impropriety of such an act would be unquestioned in any other human transaction. If a client wishes to dissociate from a lawyer, the lawyer may strongly advise against the act, but can not force the client to sign a release which implies improper behavior by the client. Forcing a patient to do so is medical blackmail.

EXCEPTIONS TO THE BASIC CONTRACT

It is necessary to acknowledge the many exceptions to the basic contract, on both individual and public levels. Recently some states have legislated the power of licensure back to public officials. The current self-care movement may be interpreted as an attempt to alter the basic contract by eliminating the physician as much as possible. In addition, there are within most countries subgroups of the population who appear to reject the established medical system and the authority of conventional physicians. In the United States some ethnic, religious and social groups either do not patronize the conventional medical system, or they do not yield full authority to physicians they do see. This is not so much a rejection of the basic contract, however, as it is a rejection of the belief system of Western medicine. These groups are usually quite willing to enter into contracts with unconventional healers more representative of their beliefs.[14]

The basic contract is firmly entrenched in most medical practices, including the unorthodox, because it is rooted in the attitudes of all societies. It is the source of each individual physician's power. Unfortunately, the power it takes away from patients and gives to doctors perpetuates most of the shortcomings of medicine.

14. These points are more fully discussed in Chapters 9 and 10.

CHAPTER FIVE

The Professional Development of Physicians

[Physician to medical student:] "I would try to convince you that my statements may be accepted, not on my humble authority, but because they are the conclusions of wise men—men wiser or certainly a little older than you, my friend—through many ages. But as I have no desire to indulge in fancy flights of rhetoric and eloquence, I shall merely say that you will accept, and you will study, and you will memorize, because I tell you to!"

> Sinclair Lewis,
> *Arrowsmith*

All professions are conspiracies against the laity.

> George Bernard Shaw

THE WAYS physicians think and behave are not natural but are the result of professionalization by the "medical subculture," which they join when they enter medical school. Although the subculture is exclusive and heavily guarded from invasion by the laity, it is as much an expression of society as art or religion. Medical schools are cultural institutions, and the way they pass on the subculture to each generation of physicians is described in the following passage:

Medical school training refines, enhances, and details the cultural role which the doctor is to play; it not only provides the student physician with the technical skills which are a part of the content of the medical sub-culture, but it also carefully sets forth standards for nontechnical action within the doctor-patient relationship. Some of the principles [the student] learns are codified in ethical terms. Many others are less formal but very pervasive attitudes and habits that are copied from clinical instructors, imposed by the expectations of teachers, patients, and nurses and/or enforced by social pressures from student peers. Habits and attitudes about how to act with patients are learned by the student physician as he adapts himself to the environment of teaching and practice. He accepts the standards and values of his preceptors, and he conforms to the accepted role of the practicing physician. The role itself is composed of those technical skills, business practices, social habits, and human relations management measures which comprise the student's picture of what a model doctor is like. Once the role, with all its technical and psychological content, is learned, it becomes a way of life. It sets the tone for the later professional behavior in the doctor.[1]

No physician can stand alone from the profession; from the beginning he is suckled by it as the babe is by the mother. He may practice alone and make decisions without consultation, but both he and his practice, especially in this day of high technology, are exceedingly dependent on the profession and interdependent with other physicians. His training conditions him to practice medicine within the tenets of the profession, and in the process, he comes to owe his first loyalty to the profession, which in turn gives direction to his clinical practices.

There are two parts of medical education, theoretical knowledge and actual practice. Before he can begin to practice, the physician must learn a scientifically oriented body of knowledge. This is the unglamorous part of medical school—books, bacteriology laboratories and medical journals. The larger part of medical training, however—application of theory and techniques to human problems—is not found in medical textbooks, but in supervised clinical practice.

PROFESSIONAL PRACTICES

The physician's clinical training reflects the opinions, predilections and interests of older doctors, with emphasis on nonmedical and nonscientific professional customs. The

1. Richard H. Blum, J. Sadusk and R. Waterson, *The Management of the Doctor-Patient Relationship*, p. 277.

student-doctor, for instance, learns to regard knowledge as a commodity that ought not to be shared with patients. Even Hippocrates cautioned his colleagues not to share medical information with patients, as doing so would only confuse them and make the task of treating them more difficult.

In nonmedical dealings it is unethical or illegal to withhold information useful to the purchaser. The medical student, whose native idealism may tell him a person has a right to know details of his own disease and treatment, actually has to learn to withhold information in deference to the professional attitude that such knowledge may frighten the patient or otherwise be harmful to him, and may make him want to participate in decisions. Thus from the beginning, students learn to subordinate the rules of normal human interactions to the tenets of the profession.

The medical student is taught to speak to patients in obscure language, a practice he might have considered unconscionable just a few years before. He first does this in the presence of teachers and peers, believing it to be a sign of maturity, and the positive response of his superiors reinforces this belief. Initially, the student is unaware of his change, being under great pressure to perform duties, attend conferences, and learn the professional standards by which he is judged. Without realizing it, he has taken the first step in responding to the needs and requirements of his profession to the detriment of his patients.

Thus, the patient's desire to go home from the hospital is subordinated to the professional need to "finish the workup." The need to get information by passing a tube into the intestines, regardless of whether such information will benefit the patient, takes precedence over the patient's wish to forego the experience. By a slow and intangible process the student learns professional discipline. The criterion becomes not what is best for the patient, but what a well-trained physician should do. The student is taught that patients' desires and opinions always must be subordinated because patients do not know as well as the physician what is best for them.

The student quickly learns on medical rounds in the hospital that his actions and words must be directed to the attending physician — that his responsibility is not to the patient, but to the physician to whom he must present the case. Upon entering the patient's room or approaching the patient's bed the student faces the attending physician, often turning his back to the patient and speaking sotto voce to prevent the patient from hearing the discussion. Occasionally a student will begin his presentation without speaking to the patient or even having eye contact with him. Through this formative ritualistic experience the student is taught that professional needs and conveniences take precedence over those of the patient. The waitress-in-training is judged by how well she serves the customer; the physician-in-training is judged by how well he serves the profession. This professional perspective allows such behavior as bringing a patient before an audience of physicians and, without so much as an introduction, proceeding with a public physical examination. Such acts run counter to normal social interchanges, and the fact that they are commonplace in hospitals shows how totally physicians take the primacy of professional needs for granted.

DECISIVENESS AND THE ELIMINATION OF SELF-DOUBT

Very little in medicine is predictable or certain. For a clinical problem presented to five clinicians there are likely to be five different suggested courses of action. As George Bernard Shaw put it:

> The very best medical opinion and treatment varies widely from doctor to doctor, one practitioner prescribing six or seven scheduled poisons for so familiar a disease as enteric fever where another will not tolerate drugs at all; one starving a patient whom another would stuff; one urging an operation which another would regard as unnecessary and dangerous; one giving alcohol and meat which another would sternly forbid, &c., &c., &c.: all these discrepancies arising not between the opinion of good doc-

tors and bad ones (the medical contention is, of course, that a bad doctor is an impossibility), but between practitioners of equal eminence and authority.[2]

The individual physician is limited not only by the fact that biomedical knowledge is incomplete, but also by his inability to learn and retain the enormous amount of knowledge on all medical subjects that does exist. There is not a clinical setting in which the physician may assume with certainty what will happen: The patient with an apparently uncomplicated common cold may in reality have lung cancer, and penicillin given to the child with an ear infection may cause death. No diagnostic test is a hundred percent accurate, and no treatment is a hundred percent effective. In many areas of medicine the likelihood of accurately predicting the course of a disease or a patient's response to therapy is little more than fifty-fifty. The clinician is constantly faced with uncertainty about whether the patient will survive, and if so, how long.

Despite the inherent uncertainty in all aspects of clinical medicine, it is rare to find a clinician who professes doubt about what is happening or what should be done. This remarkable characteristic is as old as clinicians, and is no less evident today than during antiquity. The physician speaks to the patient and the family in a voice allowing of no doubt, usually expressing recommendations for therapy as dicta which preclude appeal. Nor is doubt admitted to colleagues. The physician who expresses uncertainty is considered unknowledgeable by his peers.

Even when there is controversy over a specific test or therapy, the physician is decisive about its application to a particular patient. It is commonplace for a physician to seek opinions of consultants or colleagues about a suggested therapy, and after receiving conflicting opinions of what should be done and vacillating privately, to finally announce the decision with papal

2. George Bernard Shaw, *The Doctor's Dilemma*, p. 13.

authority. Once the decision is made, contrary suggestions or opinions are rejected, and frequently the dissenting consultants or colleagues will join in the affirmation, or at least desist from opposition which might undermine the certainty. Lingering doubts are never betrayed to the patient or family, who always perceive the decision as "the only possible one." Alternative therapies are rarely discussed with patients, as to do so would introduce doubt. Sometimes elaborate precautions are taken to preserve the appearance of unanimity in the decision, and a "united front" is presented by all associated nurses, residents and even social workers.

Only when the proposed action is obviously unlikely to succeed—as in last-resort surgery for a patient who is dying from an incurable disease—is the clinician apt to express uncertainty. He does it then to admit to his colleagues that he does not expect success, and to prepare the family for failure. When the clinician thinks there is a reasonable chance of success, he expresses no doubt at all.

Decisiveness becomes more pronounced with status. Medical students may freely express uncertainty to each other, but they rapidly learn not to divulge the feeling to their superiors who may view it as weakness as well as ignorance. The medical student who speaks with authority is considered more mature by the clinical teachers, although he dare not be inaccurate too often. The emphasis on certitude encourages answers when the student has none, including bluffing and outright lies. A dull resident will always outscore a brilliant student on rounds, not because he knows more, but because he knows how to speak authoritatively. Similarly, it is said that the difference between a consultant and a general practitioner is not in knowledge, but in the conviction with which it is spoken.

In keeping with rank, the strongest certainty tends to come from those who must make the most momentous decisions. Surgeons such as those who performed heart transplants in the glory days before the operation was abandoned by all but a few careful researchers sometimes reach the point where they are, as Denton Cooley put it, "vaulted into [a] sort of orbit" that makes them almost impervious to the uncertain nature of the act.[3]

Why, then, surrounded by the reality of clinical uncertainty, is the clinician taught to be so free of doubt? The usual answer is that the surgeon faced with an emergency can not engage in Hamletlike irresolution; he must move immediately and decisively, since hesitation could mean a fatal delay.

But this explanation rings hollow, because physicians making nonemergency decisions show this same decisiveness. The internist prescribing one antibiotic instead of another, after considering the decision for four hours, speaks as authoritatively as his surgeon colleague. Admittedly, uncertainty can postpone action, but most surgeons have plenty of time to think through the problem, if only during the five- or ten-minutes hand-scrubbing before entering the operating room. An honest physician should be able to accept uncertainty while responding to the need for action in a true emergency. The belief that decisiveness itself saves lives is an oversimplification, an idea more suited to the cinematic dramatization of a succession of emergencies met by swiftly moving white-coated healers than to clinical reality. The physician deludes himself by believing decisiveness insures certainty of outcome.

"Being certain is necessary for the patient" approaches the heart of the matter. The quintessence of therapy, irrespective of the specific beneficial effect of the treatment, is confidence in the therapist. Every healer of every persuasion understands the therapeutic imperative not to express doubt, for to do so would be to undermine this confidence. If the faith healer professed uncertainty about the Lord's willingness to heal an invalid, or the herbalist expressed doubt about the potency of a brew, would the patient not find less than maximum benefit in the treatment? The stronger the patient's belief, the more successful is the healing. Scientific studies of treatment with drugs and surgery

3. Renee C. Fox and Judith P. Swazey, The Courage to Fail, p. 318.

have shown a markedly lessened therapeutic effect when doubt about the benefit of the therapy was expressed before it was applied.[4] In preparation for an operation (abandoned about 1960) for relief of chest pain due to coronary artery disease, investigators told one group of patients that success of the operation was certain, while they told another group that the operation was experimental and the physicians doing it had no idea whether it would relieve chest pain. About eighty-five percent of the first group had persistent relief of pain, whereas in the second group only one in six had moderate relief.

The clinician must believe he is right, for without sufficient conviction the mask of certainty does not fit. The surest path to certitude is elimination of self-doubt, a practice at which most clinicians succeed.

The progress of the young physician in training may be measured by his self-reliance. During the first year after medical school the average trainee will seek information and advice from his superiors, but as he builds his personal fund of experience and takes on increased responsibility, his self-reliance grows in proportion to diminishing reliance on other sources of knowledge. His success in clinical matters so impresses him that he comes to believe in his capacity to deal exceptionally well not only with specific medical problems but with all human problems. With age the physician gains weight and infallibility.

A consequence of certitude is denial of the true complexity of medicine. Decisions and answers tend to be "yes" or "no," when realistically they should be "maybe," or "probably, but we really don't know." By denying uncertainty the clinician hides the true facts of the case. Even when he achieves the initial therapeutic goal, he gives the patient an inaccurate and misleading idea of what to expect from a treatment, and this may backfire if there is an unforeseen complication. The patient who is left paralyzed

4. L.H. Gliedman, W.H. Gantt and H.A. Teitelbaum, "Some Implications of Conditional Reflex Studies for Placebo Research," *American Journal of Psychiatry* 113(1957):1103.

after an elective back operation may be all the more bitter because of the certainty with which he was assured that the operation would succeed and that he had no option but to undergo it.

SIDE EFFECTS OF PROFESSIONALIZATION

Elimination of self-doubt leads the physician to think of himself as omniscient and omnipotent. Some psychologists see this well-known delusion of physicians as a defense mechanism. According to this theory, the physician has a phobia about the potential harm he may do if he makes a mistake. Since the classic means of handling a phobia is to deny it, the physician simply assumes that he is incapable of making mistakes, thereby hiding from his fear of doing so. When he does make a mistake he must rationalize it as a chance occurrence, so that he will not be rendered impotent by the fear of doing harm.

A simpler explanation is that omnipotence is demanded by the traditional doctor-patient relationship. The patient needs it, and therefore the physician must supply it. The Egyptian physician-priests were successful not because of the rationality of their system, but because they offered omnipotence to their patients. Belief in magical power that can defy the normal course of events is what appealed to the sick. The doctor's air of omnipotence may be an inexcusable sin to the nurse who observes it, and it may irritate healthy persons who have no need for it, but to the sick man it gives cause for hope and confidence, the basic elements of nonspecific therapy.

The trouble with the myth of omnipotence is that it inevitably leads the physician to act as if he had powers he does not have. Thus, heart surgeons transplanted hearts with confidence and enthusiasm at a time when they had insufficient scientific knowledge to succeed. In the period preceding and immediately following the first dramatic human heart transplantation there was no dispassionate reason to expect success in the experiment, since the results of operations on animals were not good, and there was little understanding of the mechanism of tissue rejection and what was required to combat it. Yet scores of medical teams did the operation, sustained by their assumed omniscience and omnipotence. Subsequent failure did not prompt a re-examination of the omnipotence myth—the failure was blamed on specific technical limitations. In less dramatic and less hazardous ways, all physicians assume omnipotence in their particular spheres of expertise.

In order to sustain belief in their own omnipotence and omniscience, physicians must be arrogant. There is no way around it. The therapeutic relationship mandates a superior attitude in the physician in his dealings with patients. Zeus slew Aesculapius with a thunderbolt because the young physician had dared to reclaim a patient from the grave. The act of curing, which has natural origins and explanations, may not by itself constitute arrogance, as the myth implies, but the physician who believes in his own personal powers of healing takes a godlike stance.

The arrogance of some physicians is almost beyond belief. Appointments, tests, hospitalizations and even child-delivery are at their convenience. They paternalistically scold, rebuke and even verbally abuse patients for not following orders, and most of them at one time or another treat patients in a manner unthinkable in ordinary relationships. Incredibly, most patients do not perceive physicians as ill-mannered, but accept this sort of behavior as a natural part of the relationship. The professional attitude banning patients from participating in decisions or even expressing opinions about proposed acts of vital self-interest is arrogant to the core. The patient who is not directly paying the bill, and especially the welfare patient, gets more than his share of professional arrogance. For many physicians arrogance seems an essential part of a relationship in which a helpless person seeks aid from one who is granted power literally over life and death.

The physician cannot be omnipotent in the operating room if he is ineffectual in dealing with his subordinate colleagues. To maintain his preeminence as leader of the team, he must dominate nurses, physiotherapists, house staff, social workers and so on. Above all, he must remain in charge. In a profession not known for the modesty of its members, the more a physician assumes the role of the great healer, the more he becomes isolated in his arrogance, with less and less honest interaction with both patients and colleagues. One need only attend a medical staff conference or Grand Rounds to observe the inordinate degree of pompousness with which physicians deal with one another.

There are those who believe that medicine attracts persons whose personal characteristics match what is required professionally; they believe that those who are naturally pompous and overbearing are attracted to medicine as a place where they will fit in without bothersome adjustments. I do not agree. I believe the professional characteristics of physicians are superimposed on personalities no different from those of other persons. As Bernard Shaw, one of the most severe critics the medical profession ever had, plaintively said, "Doctors, if no better than other men, are certainly no worse."[5] Beneath the role of the physician is an ordinary person with ordinary values. The typical beginning medical student has humane ideals and often is critical of older physicians who appear to disregard the emotional needs of patients. It is commonplace to observe in such a student at the end of his training the very behavior he decried a few years earlier.

Maybe part of the problem is that the public, in its desire for magical healing, can not conceive of the doctor as an ordinary person. Medical schools get bright students, but not the very brightest (who go into physics or biochemistry). The brightest medical students end up in nonclinical medicine, e.g., research. Some physicians are exceedingly common and dull; within the profession they are easy to spot. But to the laity they all look the same: The patient sees the professional, not the person.

5. Shaw, *The Doctor's Dilemma*, p. 68.

MEDICAL ETHICS

To the physician, medical ethics is the code, part written and part unwritten, which regulates his professional behavior. By and large, the code of medical ethics tells the physician whether he should discuss a case with another physician, whether he should have a nurse in attendance when examining a woman, whether a fee should be charged for a service and what the appropriate fee is, what should be said to the news media about celebrated cases, what his professional relationship with a nurse should be, and so on. Medical ethics historically have consisted of rules of etiquette defining relationships among physicians and regulating the activities of the medical guild; it is the social code of conduct for the medical profession which binds it together, allows a harmonious working of its constituent members, and protects them in dealing with the public.

Despite the public understanding of the basic doctor-patient relationship, the allegiance of the physician is not always to his patient, but in varying degrees is to himself and his profession. The various written professional codes of "medical ethics" have been oriented toward professional interests and represent the public only indirectly. The first great code, the Oath of Hippocrates, was at best a statement of professional standards more concerned with propagation of the profession than with the rights of patients. There is nothing in it indicating regard for the perspective of the public, and the admonitions to keep the patient from harm and not to reveal confidential information are clearly in the best interests of physicians. As a physician ethicist has commented, "The oath's content cannot be regarded directly or by inference as an adequate statement of a patient-centered ethic."[6]

The next important medical code, which has influenced medical practice in all of the English-speaking countries, was devel-

6. C.B. Chapman, "On the Definition and Teaching of the Medical Ethic," *New England Journal of Medicine* 301(1979):630.

oped by the Royal College of Physicians of London during the sixteenth century. The college set out the duties of members in a series of statutes, some of which were in conflict with English common law. The term "ethical" was applied to statutes prescribing penalties for violations of the code, although the statutes were strictly organizational, designed to control the conduct of members of the medical guild, and had nothing to say about ethical problems concerning patients. One of the enduring legacies of the statutes was the misleading use of the word *ethical* to refer to organizational rules and regulations.[7]

The American Medical Association's first code of ethics, drawn up in 1847, was designed to aid the profession during a time when conventional medicine was only one of many groups viciously competing for patients. The code served the purpose of uniting the organization and disciplining its members, and has since been revised several times. In 1957, the "Ten Principles of Medical Ethics" supplemented the more detailed "Code of Medical Ethics," but both were still primarily organizational codes that reflected changing social patterns and did not address the real questions of medical ethics and the interests of patients, except to reiterate the paternalistic concept that the physician knows what is best for the patient.

The most recent version, adopted by the A.M.A. in 1980, was prompted not by concern within the profession for the rights of patients, but by heightening pressure upon the association from without. Specifically, the 1980 "Principles of Ethics" was to alleviate a section of the old principles which hampered the A.M.A.'s defense position in outstanding chiropractic lawsuits. As an A.M.A. spokesman stated, "The Board of Trustees has a fiduciary responsibility to protect the assets of our membership. Legal counsel tells us that we need to change the principles."[8] Although the 1980 principles recognize the need to "modernize

7. Ibid.
8. "New Ethical Principles for Nation's Physicians Voted by AMA House," *American Medical News*, August 1/8, 1980, p. 9.

fully in keeping with changes in society,"[9] and Section IV states, "A physician shall respect the rights of patients," they are clearly a response to legal and social pressure from without. They do not reflect a commitment to alter professional attitudes or to change the inequality of the doctor-patient relationship. They are profession-centered, not patient-centered.

As an example of the professional redefinition of the word *ethical*, both the British Medical Association and the A.M.A. vigorously opposed contract medicine (in which there is pre-payment by the patient for health services, and the physician works for a salary) on the grounds that the practice was "unethi-cal." Unethical by whose standards? Prepayment for medical services is now common practice in the United States, and is the norm under the British National Health Service. By opposing the practice as "unethical" the medical associations identified ethics with professional self-interest rather than with a concern for the well-being of patients.

In none of these codes do we find concern with upholding the patient's rights to truth in doctor-patient interaction. To put it more bluntly, there is no mention of the true ethical questions arising from the practice of medicine.

By the process of professionalization the physician becomes secured to the rules and norms of the profession. He looks to the profession, not to the patient or to the public, for his instructions and standards. The doctor-profession relationship is as impor-tant to him as the doctor-patient relationship, perhaps more important, for ultimately, power to direct medical practices rests with the profession, not with the public. Even in the eyes of the law the physician is judged not by what happens to a patient, but by whether he adheres to professional standards. This is why almost all medical students sooner or later give up their indi-viduality and idealism and conform to professional standards. Professionalization is the social mechanism by which physi-

9. Ibid., p. 4.

cians institutionalize themselves as the ultimate source of healing power, and unite with other physicians in an effective and profitable social and economic organization.

A profession, one must quickly add, serves many useful and necessary purposes, such as codifying and transmitting knowledge, but any profession develops an interest in protecting itself. As Shaw said, "All professions are conspiracies against the laity." Accoring to the basic contract, the medical profession is surrogate protector for the public, and public interest becomes easily confused with self-interest. The change occurs in the development of the physician with the unrecognized, unspoken and barely perceptible transition from being patient-oriented to being profession-oriented.

CHAPTER SIX

Science vs. Clinical Judgment

> When one accepts one theory and rejects another that harmonizes
> with the observed phenomenon just as well, it is obvious that he
> does not follow the path of scientific inquiry, but has recourse to
> myth.
>
> Epicurus

BECAUSE modern medicine is based on information and techniques obtained through scientific means, most people assume physicians are scientists and use scientific methods. This is incorrect. There are two reasons for this mistaken belief.

First, the public does not differentiate between biological researchers—who have developed antibiotics, built artificial pacemakers, and unraveled the mysteries of chromosomes—and clinical physicians, who traditionally have applied whatever tools are available in an unscientific manner. Second, there is confusion between science and technology. Researchers use scientific methods in creating technology; practitioners use unscientific methods in deciding how to apply it. The politicians who make decisions about military strategies or nuclear power plants are not scientists just because they are dealing with technology, and the public makes a very serious mistake in thinking that physicians are scientific because they use instruments born from science. Decisions to perform diagnostic procedures and apply therapies, and methods of assessing the value of medical practices are determined by the attitudes of physicians, and these attitudes are not inherently scientific. There are, to be sure, some scientific persons who practice medicine, but the majority of physicians do not apply the fruits of science scientifically at all.

In medical school, knowledge is imparted by pronouncement, first because the student is deluged with so much biological information to memorize that he can not stop to question what he is told, and second because the medical subculture uses *ex cathedra* statements as a matter of course. Once students advance to clinical training in hospitals, they are surrounded by clinicians and peers whose interest is professional, not scientific, so that although they have learned biological principles from their textbooks, they are not taught how to apply them scientifically to clinical problems. They learn the biological causes of peptic ulcers and the biochemical effects of drugs used in treating them—how the drugs alter the ulcer physiologically—but they apply and assess the treatment the same way the ancient Egyptians did.

Students are not taught the techniques of information gathering and problem solving, the rules of evidence and inference from data, the need for controlled studies and epidemiological studies for assessing the real effects of therapies, or the fundamental fact that human responses to therapies can be predicted at best only as probabilities.

No one tells the student of the uncertainties of clinical medicine, of the absence of sufficient knowledge to make well-informed decisions in many cases, of the ease with which observations may deceive if they are not properly checked, of how the physician's own interests may conflict with those of patients. With clinical judgment as the source of knowledge, and pronouncement as the means of transmitting it, the major influence of medical school is professional, and in the process students are molded by professional interests. Scientific interests become secondary to, or a means of obtaining, professional goals. Although physicians work within a scientific belief system, and so create the appearance of being scientific, their practice is pseudoscientific.

THE SCIENTIFIC METHOD

> "He is the only revolutionary, the authentic scientist, because he alone knows how little he knows."
>
> > Dr. Max Gottlieb,
> > in Sinclair Lewis's
> > *Arrowsmith*

> The tragedy of science is that frequently a beautiful hypothesis is slain by an ugly fact.
>
> > Aldous Huxley

Science may be defined as knowledge obtained by the scientific method. The aim of science is to discover the causes of *natural* processes. Science is not judgmental; it is based on the fundamental human desire to understand the universe. Its ultimate goal is to develop a body of facts that satisfactorily explain natural phenomena so as to predict accurately and consistently the course of natural events. In medicine, scientific facts, as first introduced by the Hippocratic physicians, concern illnesses and therapies, and the conclusions drawn from the facts are used in clinical practices.

The scientific method has four parts: statement of the problem, formulation of a hypothesis, testing of the hypothesis, and conclusions drawn from the testing. The formulation of hypotheses is the most inexplicable of these parts, for hypotheses can come from any source. In the course of living, every person generates ideas, whether by intuition, messages from God or the supernatural, or observations of natural phenomena. Those who deride science as having a Procrustean disregard for paranormal insights are incorrect; indeed, under the scientific method, the wildest idea is a legitimate hypothesis, but any hypothesis must be subject to testing of its validity.

If one were to accept ideas as facts, that would be the end of it, and there would be no means of determining their accuracy. In medicine, most opinions have historically been incorrect. The marvel of the Greeks was in realizing how uncritical acceptance of seemingly rational ideas resulted in a preponderance of inaccuracies and mistaken conclusions. The answer, which is the heart of the scientific method, is to take ideas as hypotheses only, subject to verification by rigorous testing.

The truthfulness of a hypothesis can be more vigorously asserted the more vigorously it is tested, and the all-important act of science is finding a hypothesis capable of standing up to testing without being disproven. Testing is the major step in avoiding false conclusions. But testing itself must be subject to scrutiny. The investigator must not view the experimental phase as an inconvenience necessary to substantiate his hypothesis, but must freely accept the risk that the testing may disprove the hypothesis.

The crucial and exacting step that the scientist must take is to attempt to disprove his own hypothesis, and to invite others to do the same. To do otherwise is to risk the delusion of infallibility. If Galen had tried to disprove his theories about anatomy, instead of reinforcing them with reasoning, he would have recognized his mistakes and saved the world fifteen hundred years of incorrect medical thinking. The scientist must recognize his inability to be an impartial judge of his own ideas, and must exclude his own feelings and aspirations from the testing process, since they could distort his own conclusions and misdirect experimenters who attempt to confirm the work.

The scientist must learn the meaning of coincidence and probability. As noted earlier, the first physicians made the mistake of *post hoc, ergo propter hoc* when use of a particular therapy coincided with improvement of the patient. By experimental methods the scientist eliminates the confounding effect of coincidence. Failure to do so is an error as serious as any other in testing. The scientist also must understand that when dealing with medical phenomena, where absolute knowledge is rare and results of treatment are unpredictable, conclusions can be expressed accurately only in terms of probabilities.

If testing is the heart of the scientific method, drawing conclusions is the spirit of it, for logical inference from accumulated facts is the end product of science. Always the scientist must return to method, which is central to consideration of admissible conclusions. The skill is in concluding nothing more than the facts warrant. As Whitehead and Bronowski describe it, the method is repetitive—submitting conclusions to testing, modifying the conclusions, going back to more testing and more discoveries, which lead to new conclusions, and so on.[1] In the scientific process no conclusion may rest, since inferences may be distorted by the testing technique. Inquiry does not stop after the first pass; it must never stop. Nothing is final; certitude is a false luxury, for it would terminate the process and stop us where we are. Continuous testing is at once the major difficulty and the most useful tool of science, for although certainty is the backbone of most medical practices, it is destructive of scientific inquiry. The greatest responsibility of the scientist is to search for additional facts. Failure to gather more facts when it is possible to do so is a rejection of the scientific method.

In the end, science is a method of checking the belief systems that are the rational creations of man. It is not intended as a replacement for beliefs, but as a means of assessing them against the facts of the natural world.

THE CLINICAL METHOD

> Of course everyone is free to prefer his favorite article of faith to the scientific, that is the empirical method. But do not let us imagine that this faith is then anything except a piece of comfortable and customary superstition.
>
> J. Bronowski,
> The Common Sense of Science

1. Alfred North Whitehead, Science and the Modern World, p. 3; J. Bronowski, The Common Sense of Science, p. 30.

The methodology of modern clinicians is philosophically in line with Paracelsus, advanced beyond Aristotle, dangerously close to Galen, and behind Roger Bacon, Galileo, Vesalius and the mainstream of scientific thought thereafter. It is most nearly akin to that of Descartes. Descartes held that there are certain fundamental ideas gained by intuition that provide the surest starting point for deductions about the natural world. Unlike Francis Bacon and Galileo, who used experimentation to determine principles, Descartes used experiments as a means to illustrate principles already deduced through intuition.[2] The Cartesian principle that the mind and body can be treated separately, in contrast to the holistic concept of health as a state of harmonious integration of the person within himself and with his surroundings, is the philosophical keystone of modern orthodox medical thinking. But the most important influence of Descartes was his reliance on intuition as the source of knowledge. Modern medical clinical practice has not evolved beyond this stage. As a whole, physicians have never adopted the philosophical principles of Newtonian physics; the probabilistic concepts of modern physics are totally alien to them.

The clinician is predominantly an empiricist in that he bases his medical opinions on observations and experience but generally rejects scientific testing of these opinions. Modern physicians regularly attribute their patients' responses to therapies without taking into account natural recoveries or variations in illnesses. Physicians do not have a systematic method for classifying facts of illness and treatment so as to be able to say a particular treatment was definitely responsible for a particular recovery. As a rule, they believe the benefits of medical practices are self-evident, and therefore do not require testing. Clinicians traditionally accept as authority the word of noted physicians or pronouncements in medical journals. Most physicians lack a doubting, critical spirit in assessing their practices; they do not

2. Steven F. Mason, *A History of the Sciences*, pp. 166, 203.

eliminate their own biases from the process of evaluation; and their inferences are commonly based on incomplete information, hearsay evidence and unsubstantiated assumptions. They rely not on science but on intuition and clinical experience.

Clinical experience is inherently subjective and interpretive. The physician's observations are colored by his and the patient's subjective response to therapy, by the physician's interpretation of physical examinations and laboratory reports, and by the opinions of consultants. Clinical experience is limiting, for an individual physician's range of cases is necessarily narrow, given the extreme variability of human illnesses. It is a chance process, acquired sequentially (not all at once), so that early observations influence interpretations of later ones, and the physician tends to rely on a fallible and interpretive memory that selects out what seems to be important and discards what seems to be unimportant.

The physician thinks of individual cases, not of universal rules, and is confronted always with responsibilities to individual patients, not to groups of patients. He perceives that he alone is responsible for and knows the facts of the case with which he is dealing, and therefore he must rely on his own experience rather than on the collective experience of thousands of others as recorded in the medical literature, or on a body of scientific knowledge. Scientific evidence bearing on a case becomes subordinated to the physician's interpretation of that evidence. He regards scientific evidence as too general to apply to individual patients — as incomplete if not incompatible with his own evaluation — and he disregards it if it does not confirm his own experience. He will even reject statements and policies of medical societies and institutions if they do not conform to his personal experience.

Clinical experience produces "knowing," which, in most clinical practice today, is the primary means of decision making. Observation and interpretations can be wrong, and harmful practices based on such errors are incorporated into medical practice. Often years or decades of using a worthless or harmful therapy are based on insufficiently tested "knowing." One need only reflect on how fervently physicians "knew" that radical mastectomy was the best method of treating breast cancer, until after seventy years of the treatment, scientific testing challenged the claim. One cannot dismiss the clinical observations and judgments that have led to worthwhile discoveries, but the good that comes from this process of knowing without testing has always been overrated by profession and public alike, while the mistakes go unnoticed and unreported.

The average physician may bow to professional standards or peer pressure, but almost always he will choose personal opinion over scientific evidence in making clinical decisions. Consider this statement by a surgeon who spoke against subjecting appendectomy to computer analysis to determine its value: "I could not fail to operate on a patient I felt had acute appendicitis, even if there was evidence the outcome is the same without an operation."[3] This is an almost universal attitude among physicians, and is based on the common myth that the physician is somehow imbued with a mysterious sense derived from training and experience. In reality, the methods used by clinicians in problem solving are no more mysterious or difficult than those used by other people. There is no such thing as a special intuition given to the physician but denied to other ordinary persons.

The process whereby the physician uses his training and experience to formulate medical decisions is called, within the profession, clinical judgment. Sound clinical judgment is the most revered of professional traits. When there is not enough information on a case to provide a clear answer, and no time to gather the information—as in a surgical emergency—clinical judgment is necessary and useful. More frequently, however, clinical judgment is substituted for scientific knowledge. Under the rubric of clinical judgment the physician is allowed to make

3. Howard H. Rich, "How Much Government Control Do We Really Need?" *Drug Therapy* 8(1978):7.

the most serious medical decisions by the authority of his pronouncements alone, as long as he conforms to the standards of
the professional community. Unlike the architect or the en-
gineer, the physician need only demonstrate judgment for the
approval of the public and his colleagues.

To be truly scientific the physician would have to subordinate
clinical judgment to an impartial and impersonal body of
knowledge. As was the intention of the Hippocratic physicians,
personal experience would be but one step in the gaining and
storing of information. But in so doing he would lose authority,
exclusivity and mystique, and would have no more claim to
special status than the auto mechanic or the repairman. Clinical
judgment, which is inherently individual and intuitive, is incompatible with the scientific method which relies on universal,
not individual, rules. Clinical experience and clinical judgment
as the sources of knowledge in medicine are necessary if the
physician is to retain his special status, which is why they
remain central to medical practice.

TESTIMONIALS

One unscientific method of assessing the results of therapies
and other clinical practices is the testimonial, which the physician very often uses the way quacks do. As discussed in Chapter 3, testimonials are worthless and in fact misleading when
used to assess the effects of a medical practice or therapy. Case
reports, as they are called within the profession, are useful for
describing the variability of illnesses and responses to treatment, but they do not cover the full range of responses, or even
suggest the most probable ones.

The real problem with testimonials is that they are a source of
error in medical practices when they are used selectively to
promote a favored therapy. In this way, they are like testimonials
in television advertisements and faith healer meetings. The
natural tendency of physicians is to select and to believe those
testimonials supportive of their opinions. All the prehistoric

mistakes of not accounting for natural changes and psychological influences are incorporated into the testimonial, and the
common belief of both physicians and the public that multiple
testimonials strengthen the claim only compounds the error. Ten
thousand testimonials to a cure of the common cold by a patent
medicine are no more evidence than the claim made by only one
person. Hippocrates surely would be pained to see the single-
case testimonials appearing regularly in our medical journals
under the guise of scientific evidence, demonstrating that in
twenty-four hundred years clinicians have not regained the
Greek knowledge that in order to avoid the deception of the
testimonial one must study all cases. Paradoxically, although
physicians steadfastly defend the principle of individual variation and the need for individual treatment, they accept without
blinking the testimonial of one patient as evidence for treatment
of a different patient.

STATISTICS: VALUE AND MISUSE

The great variation and unpredictability of human responses
to therapy necessitate the use of statistics to formulate accurate
predictions in medicine. Very few physicians enjoy working
with statistics, and the average layman may find the subject
boring, but use of statistics is absolutely essential to the proper
conduct of modern medicine. First, because of biological variations, all medical knowledge is statistical. There are no universal laws or formulas by which the proper course of treatment can
be determined, but only probabilities based on statistical relationships of recorded observations. For example, if we ask
whether radiation therapy will prolong the life of a man with
lung cancer, it is impossible to give a definite answer for that
individual, but by pooling all information known about that
treatment for that disease and analyzing it statistically, we can
make a prediction. Second, virtually all laboratory tests are
based on statistical judgment of what is normal or abnormal.

The alternative to the use of statistics in medicine is clinical judgment. In facing a problem, the physician using clinical judgment says, in effect, "I can handle that problem. I've seen three, four, or maybe even a hundred cases like it, and I know what happened, and therefore I know what to do." That physician does use statistics, but only the ones he chooses. The patient is thus limited to his physician's personal statistics rather than having access to all statistics bearing on the case. Although each patient is unique, all treatment is based on predictions arrived at by using the same treatment on different patients, and the decision to use a particular treatment rests on either the physician's guess, or statistical analysis of more cases than he could have seen.

The public must become aware of the statistical nature of medical knowledge. To treat a patient without use of statistics would require discarding all medical knowledge obtained from other patients. Using a statistical approach to medicine may sound impersonal, but the better the statistics, the more accurate the prediction of any patient's response to a therapy.

It would be wrong to imply that no clinicians understand or use statistics well, but the average clinician uses statistics the way the average male medical student wears a necktie: reluctantly and resentfully. Most physicians in ordinary medical practice have virtually no understanding of the theory or proper use of statistics, and most of those at medical centers who are forced to use statistics use them incorrectly, to comply with regulations and as a means of gaining support for conclusions already drawn. Analyses of research studies reported in major medical journals show that almost seventy-five percent of the reports have unsupportable or invalid conclusions due to incorrect use of statistics.[4] These invalid reports represent the best use

4. S. Schor and L. Karten, "Statistical Evaluation of Medical Manuscripts," *Journal of the American Medical Association* 195(1966):1123; T.J. Sheehan, "The Medical Literature: Let the Reader Beware," *Archives of Internal Medicine* 140(1980):472; S.A. Glantz, "Biostatistics: How to Detect, Correct and Prevent Errors in the Medical Literature," *Circulation* 61(1980):1.

of statistics in medicine.

Clinicians make the mistake of supposing that the mere use of numbers and statistics makes an analysis objective and scientific. Impressed by modern technology enshrouded in numbers, and by the utility of and need for measuring amounts of urine or milligrams of sodium in the blood, clinicians develop a belief and commitment to numbers as a means of expressing biological states, but in so doing they confuse measurement with meaning, and precision with accuracy. Statistics can be produced to support any medical claim, as is apparent in television advertising. By using statistics without regard for how they are acquired or whether they represent fair comparisons, physicians deceive themselves into thinking that they are scientific.

There is a commonly held notion that the person who works with numbers is less compassionate than the person who works with "people," or that the doctor who uses statistics is less personal and humane. The use of statistics should not prevent the physician from responding to the patient's anguish and apprehension with as much compassion as is called for. In fact, the physician with more accurate knowledge can be more sincerely compassionate, for he does not need to cover over his ignorance and incompetence with false warmth. The art of medicine is the skillful application of the science of medicine for the benefit of patients, and not just the skillful manipulation of the patient's mind so as to produce a healing atmosphere. The most humane practice of medicine involves the proper mix of science and compassion, of bio-physical knowledge and concern for feelings, and the one need not interfere with the other.

ASSESSMENT OF THERAPIES

In no aspect of clinical medicine is the use of the scientific method more needed or less in evidence than in the assessment of therapies. Historically, doctors have enthusiastically embraced therapies which ultimately turned out to be of no benefit to their patients, and there is evidence of the same today. More

than one-half of widely used new surgical operations introduced during the period 1964-72 were not an improvement over
existing forms of therapy, while some were actually harmful.[5]
Recent therapies that were widely used for years or decades but
are now considered to be worthless or harmful include pure
oxygen for premature babies, chelation treatment for arteriosclerosis, intestinal bypass operation for obesity, arterial
implants for coronary artery disease, stomach freezing for the
treatment of duodenal ulcer, clofibrate[6] for arteriosclerosis, radical mastectomy for cancer of the breast, electroshock therapy for
mental illness, a series of operations for duodenal ulcer, diethylstilbestrol (DES) for pregnancy problems, prefrontal lobotomy
for mental disorders, and tonsillectomy as a routine for
everyone.

Because of the variability of biological responses, the physician almost never can state the result of a therapy or medical
practice with mathematical precision, but he can only speak of
the effect in terms of *comparison* to how the patient would have
been without the therapy. Moreover, because of natural healing
and natural variations of illnesses, it is almost impossible to say
with certainty what specific effect a particular therapy had on a
particular patient. One can not scientifically test a therapy as an
object separated from the patient, as one can test a bridge design
or a law describing the movement of the stars. A therapy does not
always work, or always not work, but it works for some patients
and not others, and there are variations in how effective it is

5. J.P. Gilbert, B. McPeek and F. Mosteller, "Progress in Surgery and Anesthesia: Benefits and Risks of Innovative Therapy," in *Costs, Risks, and Benefits of
Surgery,* ed. John P. Bunker et al., p. 142.

6. This drug, which lowers the cholesterol level in the blood, was widely
thought to be effective in preventing coronary heart disease. Recent controlled
studies show a twenty-five percent higher overall mortality rate in patients
taking the drug than in patients taking a placebo. The cause of the increased
mortality was not identified, but patients taking the drug had a high death rate
from heart disease as well as from other diseases. See "W.H.O. Cooperative Trial
on Primary Prevention of Ischemic Heart Disease Using Clofibrate to Lower
Serum Cholesterol: Mortality Follow-up," *Lancet* 2(1980):379.

when it does work. For this reason, medical practices or therapies can not be judged accurately by their effect on an individual, but must be assessed by their effect on large groups. For instance, if one patient with a heart attack is given a new therapy, we can say little about its effect, because most patients recover anyway. But if we give the new therapy to a large number of patients with heart attacks, the individual variations balance out, and we get a better picture of the net worth of the therapy. But still, we can judge the new therapy only by comparison to what would have happened without it. Always a comparison is necessary for a scientific conclusion. And comparisons in medicine are very difficult and complicated.

In order for any comparison to be scientific it must be both fair and complete, in accordance with the tenets of scientific testing. The comparison must allow full expression of scientific doubt; it must not be biased by the personal desires and influences of those who make it; it must take into account the possibility of coincidence; and the inferences made from it must be conditional and open to scrutiny. This is not the glamorous science that one gleans from television, or even from medical school, but it is probably the most important application of scientific principles in the practice of medicine.

There are actually many techniques of making a fair comparison to judge a therapy, but virtually all include the so-called control. In order to assess a therapy scientifically it is necessary to compare a group of patients receiving the new therapy with a group of patients receiving an old treatment, a placebo treatment or no treatment at all. The group not receiving the new therapy is called the control group, and the comparison of the groups is called a controlled study, or controlled trial. In a scientific comparison, the two groups of patients must be enough alike that any difference between the groups following treatments may be fairly attributed to the difference between the therapies, and not to differences between the groups. Put another way, if the control group and the group receiving the new therapy are so constituted as to be inherently different, one would expect a different outcome regardless of the treatments.

For example, assume that we want to test the effect of a new treatment for heart attacks, and for purposes of comparison we give one group of patients the new treatment, and another group receives the old, conventional treatment. Now, if the first group averages fifty years of age and all members have small heart attacks, and the control group averages eighty years of age and all have large heart attacks, the control group obviously will have a worse outcome regardless of therapy. Under these conditions it would be quite misleading to attribute a difference in the eventual outcome of the two groups to the difference in treatments. In a test of unequal groups, we can say nothing about the relative value of the new treatment except that we do not have evidence that it alone was responsible for the better outcome of the group receiving it. This is an example of an uncontrolled study.

The controlled study was first used in agriculture, centuries ago, to make comparisons between different breeds of grains. Adjacent fields of equal size were planted with different seeds, which were allowed to grow under identical conditions. Since everything was the same except the seed, the experiment was well controlled, and the inference that the seed producing the larger crop was the better one was sound. Probably the first controlled experiment in medicine was performed inadvertently by the surgeon Ambroise Paré in Italy in 1536. Paré had been using the conventional treatment for wounds, boiling oil, but ran out of oil one evening and was forced to substitute cold paste on some of the men. To his surprise, he found that the boiling oil treatment, which of course was very painful, was no better than the alternative treatment. Because the two groups of patients were alike except for the treatments, Paré's conclusion was scientifically sound.

The principle of the controlled study has been long acknowledged in medicine, although, as we shall see, it has not been widely used. George Bernard Shaw saw the need for the controlled experiment in medical affairs, as evidenced by this passage:

> In Shakespeare's time and for long after it, mummy was a favorite medicament. You took a pinch of the dust of a dead Egyptian in a pint of the hottest water you could bear to drink; and it did you a great deal of good. This, you thought, proved what a sovereign healer mummy was. But if you had tried the control experiment of taking hot water without the mummy, you might have found the effect exactly the same, and that any hot drink would have done as well.[7]

The case for the controlled trial was placed before the public by Sinclair Lewis, who in his 1924 novel *Arrowsmith* spoke the conscience of the scientist through professor Max Gottlieb, who said in response to any boast of success with any sort of therapy: "Where was your control? How many cases did you have under identical conditions, and how many of them did not get the treatment?"[8]

The problem for the scientist is to find a control group of patients similar to the group being treated. A relatively recent version of the controlled study, a superb English contribution, is the randomized controlled trial.[9] Much experience and testing have shown that the best method of getting equivalent groups is to assign patients to one group or the other randomly—for instance, by drawing numbers. This way, differences among patients are averaged out and the two groups become as nearly alike as is possible. Not only for purposes of comparison, but for statistical analysis of the differences between two groups, the randomized controlled trial is the most acceptable rigorous proof of the effect of a therapy.

Physicians dislike randomized controlled studies because generally they feel they "know" what is best for the patient and

7. Shaw, *The Doctor's Dilemma*, p. 65.
8. Sinclair Lewis, *Arrowsmith*, p. 42.
9. Austin B. Hill, *Statistical Methods in Clinical and Preventive Medicine*, pp. 3-9.

do not want to submit decision making to a chance mechanism. Patients also feel that random assignment to therapy is "impersonal." The resistance to controlled studies is in the attitude toward new therapies: If one assumes without testing that the therapy is beneficial, there follows an emotional distrust of randomized controlled studies. If one wants an unbiased assessment of the new therapy, controlled studies are the best means of obtaining it.

In the United States the law requires that drugs must be scientifically tested and proved both safe and beneficial, but for therapies not covered by the law, such as operations, verbal therapy, or new uses of old drugs, the predominant method of validation is clinical judgment supported by uncontrolled studies. Physicians not only fail to perform scientific testing, but collectively reject it as unuseful. The uncontrolled studies widely used are by their very nature inaccurate and potentially misleading and harmful.

The way a new therapy typically comes into use is that the clincian gets the idea that a certain treatment for a certain type of cancer, let us say, might be beneficial. Usually the physician believes from the beginning that the treatment will work, a perfectly natural human response, as a beneficial treatment would lessen human suffering and bring appropriate rewards to its discoverer. Accordingly, the physician administers the treatment to one or more patients, telling them of his personal belief that it will work. If the results are bad, the physician forgets the whole idea, but usually the combination of patient and physician hope is enough to produce good results. Remember: At first, any new therapy will almost always be judged favorably by patients and reported as successful by doctors, regardless of its ultimately proven value.

If the initial trial results of the treatment look good, the physician then seeks statistical confirmation through an uncontrolled study. I have never known a physician to seek to *disprove* the value of a favored treatment; invariably the uncontrolled study is designed to prove that it works. In the usual uncontrolled study the physician compares results for patients who have received the treatment with others who at different times and places have received other treatments, and sometimes the comparison is with what is "known"—the physician's opinion—to happen to patients with the same sort of cancer. Sometimes he compares patients he uses the new treatment on with patients he does not use it on or with patients of a colleague who does not use the new treatment. The physician collects his data and does a statistical analysis. Usually the results favor the new treatment; for example, fifty percent of patients not getting the new treatment died during the period of the study, whereas only twenty-five percent of patients getting the new treatment died. The physician then claims statistical evidence of the benefit of the treatment.

The conclusion is fallacious, however, because the control group is not similar to the group being given the new treatment. There is a natural tendency for the physician to give his new treatment to patients who would otherwise also do well, and not to give the treatment to patients who appear to be dying. If everyone getting the new treatment is young and has a slow-growing tumor, whereas those not receiving the new treatment are older and have faster-growing cancers, the new treatment will of course look good by comparison. The use of statistics to compare the groups may be mathematically correct, but it is medically incorrect and very misleading. Nevertheless, the physician takes the "evidence" as validation of the benefit of the treatment.

Unfortunately, this is the way most new therapies are evaluated, and reports of this kind of uncontrolled study can be found in almost any issue of any clinical medical journal today. One can understand reluctance to forego methods that have served the members of the profession so well over the millenia, but at the very least, lacking scientific evidence, clinicians should say, "We do not know." The Greek method of meticulous recording of all cases was more scientific than the uncontrolled studies used by modern physicians.

Failure to use scientific testing when it is available and applicable constitutes the most serious systematic error in clinical medicine. Scientifically controlled studies have legal, ethical and even official professional support. Food and Drug Administration regulations establish standards for the kind of tests necessary to demonstrate the effectiveness of drugs.[10] Upholding these regulations, the courts have ruled that uncontrolled studies are not acceptable as sources of evidence, that testimonials and "impressions" are not acceptable, and that "beliefs of physicians, no matter how fervently held, may be treacherous."[11] And yet the medical profession does not conform to these legal opinions in areas outside the new-drug law.

Ethicists repeatedly have pointed to the uncontrolled study as being less ethical than the controlled study because of its greater potential for inaccuracy. Both the Committee on Ethics of the American Heart Association[12] and a task force appointed by the Conference of Deputy Ministers of Health (Canada)[13] have stressed that controlled studies are not only possible but would be the best means of evaluating coronary bypass surgery, yet physicians have bitterly refused to accept controlled studies of this therapy. Instead we see the spectacle, at national meetings, of physicians proclaiming the benefits of coronary bypass surgery and disallowing contrary opinions. At the 1981 annual meeting of the American College of Cardiology a cardiologist proclaimed that "The time has come to suppress the use of controlled studies, and all criticism of coronary bypass surgery."

10. Food and Drug Administration Act of 1962, Title 21, no. 314.111, pp. 105-107.

11. Weinberger, Secretary of Health, Education, and Welfare, et al. v. Hynson, Westcott & Dunning, Inc. (1972), United States Reports 412: 609-39.

12. "An Ethical Consideration of Large-Scale Clinical Trials in Cardiovascular Diseases," report of the Committee on Ethics of the American Heart Association, Circulation 52(1975): pages 5-9.

13. "Coronary Artery Surgery," Canadian Medical Association Journal 117(1977):451-59.

To summarize: Science plays a limited role in the actual practice of clinical medicine. The clinician, who applies biological knowledge to the problems of patients, does not apply it scientifically, but subjectively. He uses the technical fruits of science but resists its method, which would challenge the supremacy of his clinical judgment and reduce him from a godlike figure to a medical technician.

How could science best be used in medicine? First, science can not replace comforting and caring, major roles of the clinician. It can not totally replace clinical judgment, for there will always be times when there is not enough information from which to make the best decision. Science thrives on imagination and intuition, so clinical experience will remain the primary source of new ideas in medicine. But it is no longer sufficient to practice on the basis of "I know what is best" or "in my experience . . . ." The good clinician should recognize the limitations of his experience and use science to test his observations and validate his practices.

Science should be used to establish the rules of evidence, given the uncertainty of medical processes and the fact that conclusions are never absolute but are at best probabilities. Science can maximize the collection of information in a modern computer data bank analogous to the meticulous recordings of the Hippocratic physicians. The role of science in medicine is to supply the clinician with more knowledge and truth so that he may better serve his patients. Ultimately, science makes the practice of medicine more humane. The good clinician will not be afraid that science will usurp his power, but will use science to enhance his ability to help sick people.

CHAPTER SEVEN

Overtreatment and the Capacity to Harm

> "It is in that way that hard-working medical men may come to be almost as mischievous as quacks," said Lydgate rather thoughtlessly. "To get their own bread they must overdose the king's lieges; and that's a bad sort of treason, Mr. Mawmsey—undermines the constitution in a fatal way."
>
> George Eliot,
> *Middlemarch*

> I firmly believe that if the whole materia medica, *as now used,* could be sunk to the bottom of the sea, it would be all the better for mankind,—and all the worse for the fishes.
>
> Oliver Wendell Holmes

> *Primum non nocere* ["First, do no harm"].
>
> Hippocrates

DESPITE THE public's firm belief in the benefits of our medical system, there is increasing opinion among persons attempting to assess health care that the net value of encounter medicine (individual physicians treating individual patients) may be negative—or if positive, minimal. Sociologists, government analysts and even some physicians have concluded that the harm done by overtreatment and overuse of technology may exceed the benefits of modern medical care, especially in hospitals.[1] This idea may be a rather large pill to swallow, but it can not be dismissed just because most of the medical profession and the public disbelieve it. At issue are the health and welfare of us all.

1. Ivan Illich, *Medical Nemesis,* pp. 3-27; Rick J. Carlson, *The End of Medicine,* p. 17; Robert S. Mendelsohn, *Confessions of a Medical Heretic,* p. 114; Thomas McKeown, *The Role of Medicine,* p. 118.

There are few, if any, who would not want the benefits of modern medicine if the need arose. Encounter medicine is able to cure and keep alive as many as ten to twenty percent of the population who need curative therapy during their lifetimes, an achievement of inestimable value. The value of conventional curing is not in prolonging average longevity from seventy-five to seventy-eight years, but in reducing the number of persons who would otherwise be cut down at a much earlier age. And the major value of physicians, caring, is not estimable in life statistics. At issue is not the legitimate function of the physician, but the extent and character of physicians' practices. Too many medical practices are not of benefit to patients, or are not worth the cost. The past editor of America's most prestigious medical journal summed it up so:

> Let us assume that 80 per cent of patients have either self-limited disorders or conditions not improvable, even by modern medicine. The physician's actions, unless harmful, will therefore not affect the basic course of such conditions. In slightly over 10 per cent of cases, however, medical intervention is dramatically successful, whether the surgeon repairs bones or removes stones, the internist uses antibiotics or palliative measures (e.g., insulin, vitamin B_{12}) appropriately, or the pediatrician eliminates a food that an enzyme-deficient infant cannot absorb or metabolize. But, alas, in the final 9 per cent, give or take a point or two, the doctor may diagnose or treat inadequately, or he may just have bad luck. Whatever the reason, the patient ends up with iatrogenic problems. So the balance of accounts ends up marginally on the positive side of zero.[2]

THE DETERMINANTS OF HEALTH

There always have been critics who charged that conventional medicine is of no benefit to the public. Writers such as Molière, Tolstoy, Shaw and now Illich have suggested that the average person would be better off not having the privilege of

2. F.J. Ingelfinger, "Health: A Matter of Statistics or Feeling?" *New England Journal of Medicine* 296(1977):448-49.

seeing a physician. Physicians have brushed off such criticism as that of malcontents who may have had unfortunate medical experiences, or of writers whose social biases prevent them from understanding biological processes. In recent years, however, many physicians have advanced the hypothesis that the real gains in health do not occur in encounter medicine, and these critics are harder to dismiss.

Professor Thomas McKeown, of Birmingham, England, has most cogently presented the hypothesis that the great health gains, as measured by declining mortality rates and decreased prevalence of diseases, are due not to physicians treating patients after they become sick, but to what are really public health measures that, by improving living conditions, prevent disease in the first place.[3] The determinants of health are nutritious food, adequate housing, enough money to buy soap and clothing, a rudimentary knowledge of personal hygiene, and an environment free of filth, worms, polluted waters, and disease-carrying animals. According to McKeown:

> If we group together the advances in nutrition and hygiene as environmental measures, the influences responsible for the decline of mortality and associated improvement in health were environmental, behavioral, and therapeutic. They became effective from the eighteenth, nineteenth, and twentieth centuries respectively.[4]

The advances in health coincided with the agricultural revolution in the eighteenth century, the industrial revolution in the nineteenth century, and the sanitary revolution in the nineteenth and twentieth centuries.

Supporting this argument is the fact that mortality rates began to decline in the last half of the nineteenth century before physicians had any effective means of combating infectious diseases, the leading cause of death. Vaccinations, beginning in the nineteenth century, played a relatively small part in reducing

3. McKeown, *The Role of Medicine*, pp. 91-118.
4. Ibid., p. 78

mortality rates when compared to improved environmental conditions, which reduced exposure to infections. As John Knowles has pointed out, even the contribution of antibiotics is small in comparison to the more fundamental preventive measures.[5]

The heroes in the health revolution were not doctors, but were sanitation engineers, politicians who saw the need for public health measures, industrialists who raised the standard of living and put money into the pockets of the workers in spite of conditions in the mines and factories, farmers who introduced new agricultural techniques, social scientists who developed and spread the new techniques of hygiene, and medical researchers who uncovered the knowledge necessary for common understanding of methods of preventing disease. The role of the practicing physician in all this was minimal; he may have helped to disseminate public health information, but as often as not his practical knowledge of sanitation measures was as inaccurate as that of the public he was treating, and his interest remained fixed on specific therapies, which were of little or no benefit to the population as a whole.

One might argue that it was the clinicians working on the front lines with patients who discerned the really important problems, and who in turn influenced medical researchers and politicians to take steps for the greater public good. No doubt observant and thoughtful clinicians did realize the futility of applying nineteenth-century nostrums to people living in squalid conditions, and were able to bring pressure on authorities to institute sanitary reforms. And we must always remember the reciprocal relationship between clinicians and researchers, each dependent on the other for information necessary to their task. The researchers who developed specific cures—the vaccines and later the antibiotics—never could have approached the problems of infection without the input of clini-

5. John H. Knowles, ed., *Doing Better and Feeling Worse*, p. 57.

cians. Still, the argument goes, these contributions of clinicians were a byproduct of personal medicine, which has played little part in the great advances of medicine over the last two centuries.

Despite the improved methods of diagnosis and curing accessible to the modern physician, most of the good health of persons in developed countries even today is due not to the intervention of clinicians, but to environmental and behavioral measures.[6] A recent U.S. Government report attributed more than fifty percent of premature deaths to unhealthy behavior or lifestyle and twenty percent to environmental factors.[7] Statistically, for example, it is almost certain that a cigarette smoker can do more to prolong his life and improve his overall health by stopping the cigarette habit than by getting the best personal medical attention available.

Genetic factors, environment and lifestyle are more important than medical services when one looks at the health of entire populations. It is well known that for males aged forty-five to fifty-four the death rate in the United States is almost double the rate in Sweden. The difference is not found in the quality or quantity of medical services, but in genetic makeup, environment and personal behavior. If chances of survival were improved by individual medical treatment by physicians, Christian Scientists should, as a group, have a lower survival rate than others in the same areas, but there is no evidence to suggest that they do. Christian Scientists benefit from public health measures, they may have better health habits, and they certainly avoid physician-induced deaths.

THE BIOPHYSICAL APPROACH TO MEDICINE

Although unscientific in practice, modern Western medicine is almost exclusively biophysical in orientation, adhering to the

6. Ibid., p. 58.
7. *Healthy People: Surgeon General's Report on Health Promotion and Disease Prevention* (Washington, D.C.: Government Printing Office, 1979).

concept that all diseases can be explained by biophysical knowledge. Diabetes is due to a lack of insulin, arthritis is a degeneration of joints, and even schizophrenia may be due to biochemical abnormalities in the brain. While these theories may be correct—and certainly scientific investigations have given us remarkable knowledge of human biology—the clinical consequence of the biophysical approach is that the patient is regarded as a machine with mechanical disorders that can be fixed by physical or chemical treatments.

The patient who goes to the doctor with chest pain becomes the case of coronary artery disease; the patient who is hyperactive becomes the case of hyperthyroidism. After a night on call one physician can tell another, "Last night I got a gall bladder, two infarcts and a carcinoma of the lung." The clinician does not think in terms of the *patient's* problem, but in terms of what is mechanically or chemically wrong. Consequently, the physician's efforts may not be in the best interests of the patient, as is demonstrated by the following example.

A patient entered the hospital with severe chest pain, and a heart attack was easily diagnosed by an electrocardiogram. The attending cardiologist ordered morphine to relieve the chest pain, and left orders with the nurses to call him if there was no improvement. When the pain had not subsided within an hour, the cardiologist felt the need for more information and elected to put a tube into the patient's heart to measure pressures and the rate of blood flow. The nurses pleaded with the cardiologist to first use more morphine, pointing out that placing a tube in the heart undoubtedly would create considerable anxiety for the patient. The cardiologist replied that it was not something he liked to do, but something he had to do in order to know how to treat the patient.

While the nurses were getting ready for the procedure, the patient's chest pain gradually diminished but did not disappear entirely. When the cardiologist told the patient what he intended to do, the patient begged to be left alone, and his chest pain began to increase. During the insertion of the tube through an incision the patient's heart fibrillated, requiring an electrical shock to bring it back to normal. The procedure took about an hour, during which time the patient had continuous chest pain that went away only after the procedure was over and he was left alone.

This is an example of what can happen when the physician thinks not of the patient and his illness, but of the disease and how to measure it. What the patient needed was relief of pain, which he could have got from rest and reassurance. But the physician's training compelled him to get as much information as it was possible to measure, in the belief that only with maximum knowledge of what was happening mechanically could he treat properly. "The doctor is treating himself" refers to this kind of behavior, emphasizing that the physician is satisfying his own needs without regard for those of the patient.

"Treating the lesion" is another way of putting it. A lesion is an abnormal structural change of a diseased part of the body. In coronary artery disease, lesions are narrowings of the arteries supplying blood to the heart. It is now common practice to perform heart surgery to "bypass" such lesions even when the patient has no illness, i.e., no chest pain or disability. Even in cases where there is no evidence that such surgery prolongs life or prevents heart attacks, physicians often recommend operations in order to correct the anatomic abnormality. This is not scientific medicine, even though it utilizes scientifically derived techniques. It is philosophical medicine, based on the belief that treating abnormal mechanical structures is always proper, despite a lack of supporting evidence.

Once an abnormality is found, professional beliefs and standards compel the clinician to treat it. If a patient's blood sugar is abnormally low, the physician will treat the low blood sugar, notwithstanding the fact that the patient may always have had it and has always functioned well with it. The cardinal sin of the physician is to allow a patient to die "out of balance." "The operation was a success but the patient died" is supposed to be a joke, but it dramatizes two bad consequences of this attitude: Treatment is directed at lesions, not persons, and success of treatment is measured by correction of the lesion, not by improvement in the patient's condition. There is nothing more perplexing to the physician than to have a patient whose lesion has been corrected return with the same symptoms he had before the "cure." While obsessed by anatomy and physiology, the physician becomes heedless of the patient's legitimate concerns.

Emphasis on biophysical abnormalities directs attention to disease, not to health. The patient who has no disease is of no interest to the physician because there is no abnormality, and therefore nothing to treat. Consequently, within the biophysical frame of reference there is little place for preventive medicine. Physicians do advise patients how to take care of themselves, but this is an exceptionally small part of most practices and is done mostly as a public relations gesture. The surgeon who bypasses coronary artery lesions recommends exercise and a good diet as a means of preventing heart disease as facilely as beer can manufacturers preach against littering. But by his biophysical approach to the problem the surgeon has in fact bypassed preventive medicine and has diverted the resources of the community to attacking the lesion after it has been developed, instead of preventing it. It is a cruel hoax for physicians to preach healthy lifestyles while practicing a form of medicine which encourages the quick cure rather than prevention. In most universities preventive medicine is taught in a school separate from the medical school, so that clinicians view it as distinct from the primary practice of medicine. Physicians in public health are looked down on by stethoscope-toting clinicians, who regard them as dropouts from "real medicine."

The physicochemical approach deserves credit for eliminating many dread diseases, and it is unmatched by other systems in curing diseases, but it is limited to treating physical structures and functions and disregards the elements of human illness that pertain to the psyche. It is commonly said of Western medicine—and particularly of American medicine, where the biophysical approach is practiced in the extreme—that if the patient truly has a disease, and if he is treated for that disease and no other, he will have the best chance of cure that has ever been possible. But, if the patient does not have a disease, or is treated for a disease other than the one he has, he may be worse off under Western-style medicine, especially in America.

The biophysical approach excludes emotional, social, cultural and other problems which play an important part in human disorders. The act of curing does not necessarily exclude caring, but reliance on curing tends to make the physician disregard the need for caring, even in psychotherapy. Most patients with psychosomatic disorders (physical symptoms brought on by emotional upset), are in danger of being given drug or surgical therapy that can not possibly remove the underlying cause of the disorder, and may make it worse. Consider the following case:

A man developed chest pain which both he and his physician attributed to coronary artery disease. He underwent open-heart surgery after which he had no chest pain and was listed as cured by the operation. There is reason to believe that this operation was unnecessary. The man was fifty-eight years old when his illness arose, the exact age at which his father had died suddenly of presumed heart disease. Within a week from the time he first saw a physician for the problem, two of his colleagues had heart attacks, and one of them died. The man had tremendous anxiety over the possibility of having heart disease himself, and upon being told that he had a small lesion in his heart that could be cured by bypass surgery, he was so relieved that he had no chest pain during the three weeks before the operation, despite physically exerting himself to a point that would have caused chest pain in anyone with real disease.

This case shows the potential for unnecessary treatment when only biophysical considerations are taken into account. The man's chest pain was acknowledged to be unusual for coronary artery disease, and testing before the operation did not show changes on the electrocardiogram typical of coronary artery disease. Still, the physicians, thinking only in terms of mechanical problems, blamed the pain on the small lesion when in reality it probably was due to apprehension over reaching the age at which his father died, and the shock of the heart attacks of his colleagues. Even though the patient's chest pain ceased before he had surgery, the operation was given credit for the cure. The narrowness of vision that led to incorrect therapy led also to an incorrect evaluation of the effect of the therapy. The fact that the patient himself credited the operation with saving his life only adds to the overall misconception of what happened. One of the worst limitations of biophysical medicine is its failure to view the patient's illness within the framework of his life and identity.

Biophysical medicine is not very effective for patients with chronic diseases. For those who are incurably ill, either with fatal or nonfatal diseases, caring is extremely important, which is why many patients with chronic diseases prefer non-Western healers who at least give them hope. The Western physician often loses interest in such cases. Being preoccupied with the intrigues of diagnosis and the heroics of curing, he may even resent the patient with whom he can not fulfill his goal.

The fate of the elderly is generally that of the chronically ill, with the difference that the elderly usually die with their chronic diseases. In addition to having no professional incentives to look after the elderly, there are social disincentives. Elderly people tend to be immobile; they take more time to examine; sometimes they can not hear what the doctor is saying; they are incontinent of feces and urine; and so on. In the U.S., a positive incentive to taking care of the elderly emerged with Medicare, which in effect eliminated the financial disincentive of taking patients from the group least able to pay. The nursing home has evolved as a medical solution to what is a social problem, a solution for which the public is as responsible as the medical profession, but which substitutes medical acts of curing for what should be social acts of caring.

The elderly share an increasing dependence on the medical profession that is fostered by society. This is seen in its extreme form when the patient is dying, and especially when the patient is dying in an intensive care unit within a hospital. In such units the patient is increasingly captive to instruments and machines, and the physicians who direct them.

The attitude of the physician that the death of a patient is a professional defeat, and recovery is a signal victory, is a common observation. This attitude unquestionably serves well the patient who is young, or the patient who has potential for meaningful life if he recovers, but as a fixed proposition it reflects professional values and not the considered interests of patients. If decisions as to how to handle the elderly dying were put to a panel of nonphysicians who adequately represented the wishes of patients as distinct from professional dictates, would they make a favorable judgment on the common medical practice of doing every test possible, and doing everything to extend life as long as possible, often with disregard for pain or other forms of suffering? What can be the justification, other than following professional norms, of needlessly keeping patients alive, by extraordinary means, against the wishes of the patient and the family?

It can be argued that sick and dying people act irrationally, and are incapable of making important life and death decisions. This may frequently be true, but is no excuse for the total assumption of power by the medical profession without open and honest consultation with other people who are in a position to represent the patient. The degrading acts and infliction of pain perpetrated by physicians in order to sustain life at all costs represent perhaps the lowest expression of physician allegiance to professional norms, an allegiance that is surely misguided, for not only does it rob the patient of a dignified death, but it is certain to produce hostility among the friends and family who are dispossessed by the act. The great hubris of the physician is not in his assumption of responsibility, or even in the suffering resulting from his acts, but in his expropriation of the dearest right of life, the right to control one's own destiny.

The molding of sickness activities to professional norms occurs most particularly in the place of death for most patients. Why should the patient die in the hospital, rather than at home, where it is more natural? Relief of pain is no answer, for in most cases pain can be handled at home, and for many patients pain is produced and prolonged by being in the hospital. In the hospital the family is kept away, denying the patient the greatest source of comfort and happiness. The belief mutually shared by patient and physician, that the patient needs special services available only from the physician and within the hospital, is largely a myth. Any patient who wishes to die in a hospital may certainly do so; is it too much to ask that a patient wishing to die at home may also do so? The ritual of death in hospitals has hidden for more than a generation the human experience of natural death as contrasted with the contrived and artificial hospital death where the caring of people is replaced by the inexorable harassment of machines. Dying in hospitals serves professional needs to control the relationship; it is not done from the perspective of patients. I am reminded of an 86-year-old dying woman who, after the third resuscitation within twenty-four hours, looked up and asked, "Why am I still here?" She had been robbed of the most natural event of her entire existence.

Nothing is more representative of modern medicine than the "high technology" that testifies to the belief of both the profession and the public in progress through biophysical advances. And so there appear intensive care units, radioisotope scanning, and artificial hearts as ends in themselves, with little attention paid to how we apply these remarkable technologies. What we need more than an artificial heart is the Second Coming of

Hippocrates, with a renaissance of the scientific spirit of detachment from personal beliefs, and rigorous inquiry into the real benefits of medical practices.

IATROGENIC HARM

Iatrogenic means "induced by a physician." Strictly speaking, all changes induced by physicians are iatrogenic, but in common medical usage iatrogenesis refers to *injury* that results from a physician's intervention. If a patient sees a physician and is neither helped nor harmed, the net effect is neutral. If medication gives relief from arthritis but causes an equally distressing ulcer, there is an equal balance of benefit and harm. Iatrogenesis is counterproductivity in medicine, the rendering of a patient less healthy by the ministrations of a physician.

Most people do not realize the potential for medically induced harm. Complications from medical interventions include strokes, loss of limbs, paralysis of limbs, heart attacks, kidney failure, and almost all forms of physical as well as emotional impairment. Death due to medical intervention with drugs or surgery is commonplace, although frequently the cause is unrecognized. Most iatrogenic harm is rationalized as "unavoidable," and explained away with "It would have happened anyway." The distinction between naturally occurring disease and that induced by physicians is usually unclear. Since it is impossible to know what would have been the natural course of the patient's illness, iatrogenic disease is often attributed to natural causes. The modern physician is not different from his forefathers in ascribing cures to his personal powers and relegating failures to forces beyond his control. Nor does the public usually consider iatrogenic causes when therapy fails; people die under the care of physicians every day, but malpractice suits are rare.

If *post hoc, ergo propter hoc* were applied equally from the perspectives of failure and success, the physician might be seen in a more realistic light. That is to say, if all deaths, complications and treatment failures were perceived as causally associated with physicians' acts, as successes are, there would be a more accurate perception of the healer's powers and net value. I am reminded of a patient who was brought to the hospital for treatment of a heart attack. Unfortunately, infection which developed on a tube unnecessarily inserted into the heart spread, causing him to lose both lower legs. The patient and his family cheerfully credited the doctors with saving the man's life, but did not harbor the thought that the loss of limbs was avoidable. Nor did the physicians involved acknowledge that iatrogenesis was responsible for the infection.

The concept of iatrogenic harm is infrequently discussed in public, despite its ubiquity. We read of remarkable medical cures in the newspapers daily, but rarely do we read or see on television reports of medically induced harm. Physicians themselves do not always recognize iatrogenesis.

When recognized, iatrogenesis is destructive to healing not just by its specific injury, but by its rupture of trust in the healer, which may be harder to repair. Thus, it is not surprising that iatrogenesis is not looked for by either side and therefore is not often seen. The extent of iatrogenic disease will not be known until we have standards for administering therapies and technologies, and adequate means of measuring results. Until that time, we can only document its existence and estimate its extent.

EXCESSIVE TESTING

As one physician put it, the normal person is the one who is insufficiently investigated.[8] Probably the most common setting of iatrogenesis is medical testing.[9] Doctors order most tests in

---

8. Edmond A. Murphy, *The Logic of Medicine,* p. 123.
9. Ironically, because physicians do not understand scientific processes, they acquire an unjustified belief in the results of laboratory tests. In 1975, in a sample of medical laboratories in the United States, erroneous results were

order to "gain knowledge," to screen for disease, to be sure not to miss anything, or to protect themselves against a potential lawsuit. Most physicians are unaware of the volume of blood taken for routine tests, the cost, the discomfort, and the potential harm to the patient.

The clinician's tendency to measure whatever can be measured leads to unnecessary laboratory tests. All the professional and financial incentives are in the direction of too many rather than not enough tests. Under the guise of "good practice," laboratory tests, special procedures, "blood gases," electrocardiograms, scans, catheterizations and countless other tests are ordered without a thought beyond their availability, and without respect for the cost to the patient and to the community. One well-known American physician noted "the present-day tendency towards a five-minute history followed by a five-day barrage of special tests in the hope that the diagnostic rabbit may suddenly emerge from the laboratory hat."[10]

Estimates of the amount of unnecessary testing are little more than guesses because of the difference of opinion among physicians about what is necessary and what is unnecessary. But the Subcommittee on Health of the U.S. Senate estimated that more than thirty percent of 240 million X ray procedures in 1977 (at a cost of over six billion dollars) were unnecessary.[11] This is probably a conservative estimate. A heart specialist judged that over ninety percent of electrocardiograms taken were of no benefit to either the patient or the physician requesting them.[12] One of the more senseless rituals in medicine is to order routine laboratory tests while the patient is in the hospital. An example is the test to check on the level of a blood-thinner. While the patient is in the

found in more than a quarter of all tests. (Mendelsohn, *Confessions of a Medical Heretic*, p. 6.)

10. T.R. Harrison, "The Value and Limitation of Laboratory Tests in Clinical Medicine," *Journal of the Medical Association of Alabama* 13(1944):382.

11. Office of Technology Assessment Project Proposal (78-15), Appendix B (October 1978), p. 52.

12. S.J. Reiser, *Medicine and the Reign of Technology*, p. 158.

hospital, the test is often made every day, but when he is not in the hospital, a test every week or every month seems to be sufficient. If the patient is available, that which can be tested will be tested. As a conservative estimate, approximately two-thirds of all medical tests are of no benefit to the patient.

Can excess medical testing harm patients? Unequivocally, the answer is yes. According to one study, of patients who had diagnostic testing of the sort requiring that a needle, tube or catheter be put inside the body, fourteen percent had at least one complication, and of those having a complication, over three-quarters required either specific treatment to counteract the complication or prolonged hospitalization or both. [13] Analysis of the use of a thin needle to obtain biopsies (pieces of tissue from within the body) showed a thirty-two percent complication rate, one-third of the complications being "major." [14] Most testing that requires more than taking blood or urine from a patient runs a small but definite risk of death. Having needles inserted into the body, running on a treadmill, or even having dye injected for a kidney X ray can lead to death by unforeseen complication. Deaths from testing are viewed by physicians as aberrations, accidents within an imperfect system. But in fact these deaths are due to the systematic error of overtesting. Many of these tests are extremely helpful, and some are essential, in determining curative therapy, but the risk of complication is worthwhile only when the predictable benefit is greater than the risk.

Physicians dismiss one death in a thousand tests as an "acceptable risk," but one should ask, "Acceptable compared to what?" The physician who uses a test with a ten percent risk of complication, when the chance of benefit is only five percent, is not doing his patient a favor, regardless of the emotional desire to help. Even the presumed "safe" tests (e.g., blood tests) can cause harm. Not infrequently, a patient loses so much blood from

13. S.A. Schroeder, K.I. Marton and B.L. Strom, "Frequency and Morbidity of Invasive Procedures," *Archives of Internal Medicine* 138(1978):1809.

14. "MDs Flout Warning on Thin-Needle Liver Biopsy," *Medical World News*, January 8, 1979, p. 38.

routine testing that he gets anemia.[15] Inflammation of veins or arteries from which blood is drawn also occurs. Most injuries of this type either go unrecognized or are considered inconsequential.

OVERDIAGNOSES

Physician-induced harm can originate with diagnosis, from overdiagnosis and incorrect diagnosis. Incorrect diagnosis sometimes results from incompetence but more often from incomplete or inaccurate information. Incorrect diagnosis of a disease that is actually present is usually a limited mistake. As the disease becomes worse, the correct diagnosis comes out. Incorrect diagnosis is not a systematic problem of the profession, as every conceivable inducement is for the physician to correctly diagnose disease when present. This is perhaps the soundest part of all medical practice. The systematic and recurring error, however, is in overdiagnosis, or diagnoses of diseases which are not present.

Overdiagnosis is sometimes due to the built-in error of all tests that results from the natural variation of individuals. Most laboratory tests are designed to be only ninety-five percent correct, meaning that five percent of patients said to be abnormal really are normal. In reality most tests are less than ninety percent accurate. Also, many laboratory tests require interpretation by physicians, and it is well known that with many tests, such as X rays, the intepretations of physicians vary considerably.

By the mathematics of medical testing, a normal person who has twenty or more tests has a less than thirty-six percent chance of being judged normal by all the tests.[16] As it is routine to obtain more than twenty tests when a patient first enters a hospital (with automatic machines twenty different blood tests are run on one small blood sample), most patients are reported as having abnormalities, and to the clinician abnormality is the equivalent

15. A.L. Rosenweig, "Iatrogenic Anemia," *Archives of Internal Medicine* 138(1978):1843.
16. Murphy, *The Logic of Medicine*, p. 123.

of disease. Excessive testing in people who are normal is the primary source of mistaken diagnoses.

Behind the tendency to overdiagnose is the assumption that medical diagnosis is in itself neutral and harmless in comparison to the dangers resulting from disease. But overdiagnosis can be harmful to patients in two ways: Unnecessary treatment for nondiseases carries a risk of harm, and the mistaken belief in the presence of disease results in emotional, economic and social harm. Overdiagnosis because of misinterpretation of exercise tests has sent many a patient to open-heart surgery without a real need. Overdiagnosis of pulmonary embolism, or blood clot in the lung, has led to overtreatment of thousands of patients, some of whom have not survived the treatment.[17]

Those who are well but made ill are perhaps the least recognized but most harmed by medical practices. More than a third of all children have a heart murmur. If the murmur is confused with disease, the child may suffer incalculably. In one study ninety-three schoolchildren were diagnosed as having either heart disease or rheumatic fever (which commonly leads to heart disease). Upon closer examination only seventeen were found to have heart disease. Of the children who actually had no heart disease, thirty were restricted in their activities, six of them severely so.[18] Diagnosis of dreaded diseases always incapacitates the patient, increases emotional stress, imposes dependency and economic cost, and produces an unhealthy fixation on illness. In the example given, more children were disabled by the diagnosis than were helped by discovery of the disease. Physicians are not the only ones guilty of overdiagnosis. Charitable groups that organize disease hunts may do more harm than good.[19]

17. E.D. Robin, "Overdiagnosis and Overtreatment of Pulmonary Embolism: The Emperor May Have No Clothes," *Annals of Internal Medicine* 87(1977):775.

18. A.B. Bergman and S.J. Stamm, "The Morbidity of Cardiac Non-Disease in Schoolchildren," *New England Journal of Medicine* 276(1967):1008.

19. Lewis Thomas, "On the Science and Technology of Medicine," in *Doing Better and Feeling Worse*, ed. John Knowles, pp. 43-44.

Physicians and the public alike have an insufficient understanding of the extent of overdiagnosis and the harm resulting
therefrom. The false diagnosis of syphilis harmed people for
many years. When a blood test for syphilis was introduced in
1911, it was accepted by clinicians as firm proof of the presence
or absence of the disease. It took decades for doctors to realize
that fully fifty percent or more of those with positive tests did not
actually have the disease. Meanwhile, clinicians made somber
and often sanctimonious false diagnoses that damaged the lives
of thousands of innocents because until about twenty years ago
being known to have syphilis meant social and often economic
ruin. The diagnosis of syphilis also caused needless mental
anguish to those who actually had it, for although physicians
believed it to be a devastating and fatal disease, we now know
that eight-five percent of patients who contract it and are untreated have a normal life span, and seventy percent have no
evidence of it at death. This is an example of harm caused by
failure to obtain scientific evidence for traditional medical assumptions, and failure to examine the problem from the perspective of the patient.

HARM FROM THERAPY

Since the most action in medicine is in the field of therapeutics, the tendency to overdiagnose is more than matched by the
tendency to overtreat. All professional and economic incentives
are in the direction of overtreating. It is "good practice" to treat
whenever there is any doubt of the presence of disease, whereas
it is "bad practice" to forego treatment when disease is present.

Theoretically, treatment should be most indicated when it is
innocuous and the risk without treatment is great. Treatment
should be given most cautiously when its effectiveness is minimal or unknown and the risks are great. It is a mistake to try to
"cure" most patients, and physical treatment, given for whatever
reason, amounts to "curative" treatment. As most patients visit-
ing physicians get one treatment or another, by common reckon-

ing fully eighty percent of patients do not need the treatment they get, ten percent of patients get ineffective curative treatment because nothing effective is available, and the other ten percent may benefit from treatment, subject to complications. If eighty to ninety percent of treatments are unnecessary, iatrogenic harm is inevitable, since intervening in the natural biological processes of the body is a way of causing trouble as well as bestowing benefit, and if there is no benefit to bestow, the odds favor harm.

The overuse of drugs is epidemic. Patients and clinicians rely on drugs to take care of almost all conceivable problems, most of which are not responsive to a pharmacologic solution. There is not a drug on the market with no adverse side effects, unless it is mountain water. Drug reactions or complications are responsible for five percent of all hospital admissions in the United States, or as many as 1,500,000 persons a year, and this represents a small part of those who are harmed by drugs.[20] Commonly used medicines predictably make people drowsy, lethargic, nauseated, impotent, fatigued; they produce rashes, ulcers, seizures, anemia, jaundice and even whole diseases. Antibiotics, notorious for harmful side effects, by one estimate are given on the basis of proper indications in only one of ten instances.[21] The potential for ameliorating illness and actually curing persons of diseases by the judicious use of drugs is enormous, but on balance it is hard to be sure that they improve the health of the overall population or of individuals. The quick-fix solution sought for emotional problems or for chronic or incurable diseases produces incalculable harm, as does the injudicious overuse of drugs when the initial use is appropriate. The only certainty in attempting to assess the overall benefit or harm from the use of drugs is that there is much more harm from them than need be, and with better standards for treatment and means of

20. Spencer Klaw, *The Great American Medicine Show*, p. 26.
21. H.N. Beaty and R.G. Petersdorf, "Iatrogenic Factors in Infectious Disease," *Annals of Internal Medicine* 65(1966):641.

assessing drug effects, this form of iatrogenic disease could be reduced substantially. My personal opinion is that if physicians wrote only one-quarter to one-third of present drug prescriptions, the public would be the winner.

Iatrogenic disease is more likely to occur in a hospital. There all the pulls and pushes of professional and economic incentives are accentuated. If only because the patient is bodily present and the physician sees him recurrently, the likelihood of unnecessary treatment is greater. If it is almost impossible for a patient to leave an office encounter with a physician without a prescription, it is more nearly impossible for him to be in a hospital without receiving major treatment. In a study reported in the *New England Journal of Medicine,* thirty-six percent of patients on a general medical service (no surgery included) of a university hospital had an iatrogenic illness. In nine percent of these patients the incident threatened life or created disability, and in two percent, the illness contributed to the death of the patient.[22] Patients should avoid hospitals whenever possible. Above all, a well person is at risk in a hospital, for the probabilities of over-diagnosis and needless treatment there are formidable.

EXCESS SURGERY

In 1973 doctors in Israel went on strike for a month, during which time they attended only emergency cases. The death rate for the country dropped fifty percent, the largest decrease in mortality since the previous doctor's strike twenty years before. In Bogotá, Colombia, in 1976, doctors were out for fifty-two days, with a concomitant thirty-five percent decline in the mortality rate. In a strike in Los Angeles, also in 1976, there was an eighteen percent decrease in the death rate during the strike period, with the death rate returning to the usual level when the strike was over. A survey of seventeen major hospitals disclosed that sixty percent fewer operations than usual were performed

22. K. Steel et al., "Iatrogenic Illness on a General Medical Service at a University Hospital," *New England Journal of Medicine* 304(1981):638-42.

during the strike period.[23] Not all of the decrease in mortality in these strikes can be attributed to decreased surgery, but some of it undoubtedly can.

Excess or unnecessary surgery is the most professionally and politically sensitive area of iatrogenesis because it concerns a specific group of physicians, surgeons. The issue is discussed with considerable emotion. Like other aspects of iatrogenic disease, the amount of unnecessary surgery is impossible to measure — primarily, because there is no agreement as to what is unnecessary and what is necessary. Many surgeons claim there is no unnecessary surgery, while other physicians feel that "somewhere around ninety percent of surgery is a waste of time, energy, money, and life."[24]

Some advocate using the terms *appropriate* and *inappropriate* instead of *necessary* and *unnecessary,* but in the end the argument hinges on one's definition of need. Is the need perceived by the patient the way it is by the physician? Does the physician really know what the patient needs, and is the patient really capable of determining what he needs? Perhaps the best definition of unnecessary surgery is that which occurs when costs exceed benefits, as assessed by a well-informed consumer who makes the choice. But the consumer is seldom well-informed, and often does not make the choice. In the last analysis, we do not know whether unnecessary surgery is common or rare, because we have no valid measurements of it. We can only look at indirect evidence, and make estimates.

There always has been unnecessary surgery, by retrospective historical analysis, despite denials at the time. Not too many years ago an operation called suspension of the uterus for retroversion (an unusual position of the uterus, thought to be a common cause of backache) was very much in vogue as was tonsillectomy, and appendectomy was done much more frequently than today. At that time surgeons and referring physi-

23. Mendelsohn, *Confessions of a Medical Heretic,* p. 114.
24. Ibid., p. 49.

cians adamantly rejected any suggestion of unnecessary surgery, and yet today we consider these operations unnecessary as done then. There is, in fact, no period during the history of medicine that later ages did not judge to have practiced unnecessary surgery, and yet physicians doing it at the time pronounced it necessary. Why would we not suspect unnecessary surgery today? The conditions for assessing surgery have not changed; those who do it evaluate it.

Some current surgical practices are controversial. Many surgeons advocate removing all thyroid nodules. If this were done routinely, the number of deaths resulting from the procedure would far surpass the lives saved by it. Some heart surgeons and their colleagues advocate coronary bypass surgery for all patients who have any narrowing of their coronary arteries, and some routinely use the operation for all patients with acute heart attacks. By the conservative standards of the profession this is unnecessary surgery.[25] Although the conclusion is disputed, many analysts note that the more surgeons there are in an area, the more operations performed, without evidence of increased need in these areas.[26] The present excess of surgeons in the United States may have created an excess of operations. If the higher number of operations in some areas were of benefit for the population, groups having more operations per capita should have a lower mortality rate. Studies of appendectomy show the opposite result: The higher mortality rates were in groups with the higher appendectomy rates.[27]

The most common method of estimating unnecessary surgery

25. J.A. Mantle et al., "Emergency Revascularization for Acute Myocardial Infarction: An Unproved Experimental Approach," American Journal of Cardiology 44(1979):1407.

26. J. Wennberg and A. Gittlesohn, "Small Area Variations in Health Care Delivery," Science 182(1973):1102; J.P. Bunker, "Surgical Manpower: A Comparison of Operations and Surgeons in the United States and in England and Wales," New England Journal of Medicine 282(1970):135; E. Vayda, "A Comparison of Surgical Rates in Canada and in England and Wales," New England Journal of Medicine 289(1973):1224.

27. J.P. Bunker and B.W. Brown, "The Physician-Patient as an Informed Consumer of Surgical Services," New England Journal of Medicine 290(1974):1051.

is comparison of practices in different areas and under different financial systems. Bunker's famous study showed a rate of surgery twice as high per capita in the United States as in England and Wales, and noted that there are twice as many surgeons per capita in the United States.[28] The difference is marked, but one can not be sure which surgical rate is closer to the ideal. As the overall mortality rates for the two countries are not different, one can at least conclude that the increased surgery in the United States does not have an effect on survival. A discrepancy is also present in the finding that the overall rate of surgery is thirty-one percent higher in the Midwest than it is in the southern part of the United States, but the mortality rates are the same.[29] Approximately twice as many operations are performed on fee-for-service patients as on those enrolled in prepaid plans. Although it is possible that patients in prepaid plans receive fewer operations than they need, there is no evidence that their health is worse than that of fee-for-service patients. A more likely explanation for the difference is that fee-for-service patients get more operations than they need. Coronary bypass surgery, overall the most lucrative operation in the arsenal, is performed on a per capita basis more than five times as often in the United States as in Western Europe, whose medical care standards and accessibility to patients equal or exceed those in the United States. In North America, the rate of coronary bypass operations performed on fee-for-service patients is approximately three times that performed on patients under prepaid plans.[30] In London, more coronary bypass operations are performed for fee on patients from the Middle East than are performed in all of Great Britain under the National Health Service.

A congressional subcommittee estimated that in the United

28. Bunker, "Surgical Manpower," p. 135.

29. "Feds Launch Drive for Second Opinions," *Health Care Week*, October 9, 1978, p. 3.

30. Thomas A. Preston, *Coronary Artery Surgery*, pp. 165, 173.

States there are annually 2.4 million unneeded operations, cost-
ing $4 billion, with a loss of 11,900 lives.[31] A 1973 study of
members of two New York unions showed a 17.6 percent rate of
unnecessary operations.[32] The independent Health Research
Group estimates a minimum of 3.2 million unnecessary operations per year, at a cost of $4.8 billion and 16,000 lives; the group
further estimates that half of all operations under Blue Cross may
be unnecessary.[33] For all these estimates, the standard of acceptable rates is set by prepaid groups.

Although we can not make accurate measurements of excess
surgery, the marked difference between payment systems
suggests that economic influences alone account for a twofold
difference in rates of surgery. Even without financial incentives
there is at least a doubling of the surgical treatment rate due to
professional and social influences (as with all sorts of therapy),
and so I estimate that about three-quarters of all operations are
unnecessary.

Physicians may disagree about whether there is unnecessary
surgery, or how much there is, but they are united in vigorous
opposition to discussion of the subject in the popular media.
Even those who think it ought to be investigated want an internal discussion, restricted to the profession, to avoid loss of
confidence by the public in the specific treatment and in the
physicians dispensing it. Physicians argue, "Why dig into all
this and upset patients who already have had the treatment, and
undermine physicians who intend to use it?"

The ardor with which physicians attack any attempt at public
discussion of unnecessary surgery shows their understanding
that the therapeutic effect of trust in the doctor is an important

31. J.E. Moss, "Congressional Scrutiny Reveals Sore Spots of U.S. Health
Care," Legal Aspects of Medical Practice 6(1978):29.
32. E.G. McCarthy, "Effects of Screening by Consultants on Recommended
Elective Surgical Procedures," New England Journal of Medicine
291(1974):1331.
33. Testimony of S.M. Wolfe, of Public Citizen's Health Research Group,
before the House Subcommittee on Oversight and Investigations on Unnecessary Surgery, July 15, 1975.

source of success of surgery. If surgery, or for that matter any therapy, could stand on its own merits, public controversy would have a negligible effect on its benefits. Open discussion will never undermine any truly beneficial therapy.

CONCEALED EXPERIMENTATION

The wise physician, it is often said, understands that every treatment is a form of experiment, because the exact response is unpredictable for each individual, but therapies that have been well tested are not experimental insofar as their probable safety and benefit have been established. Therapy remains essentially experimental until there is sufficient evidence of such probability, and there is much potential harm in the use of unproven therapies.

The Vineberg operation,[34] which was popular during the sixties, is an example of an experimental practice that patients assumed was established. It was widely performed on patients with coronary artery disease until about 1970, when the new coronary bypass surgery replaced it. Although the Vineberg operation is now considered obsolete and useless by medical consensus, an estimated 10,000 to 15,000 people underwent the procedure believing that it was a proven treatment. The fatality rate was between five and ten percent, meaning that approximately 1,000 persons died from the operation. Knowing now that this particular therapy is of no value and was potentially harmful to everyone exposed to it — not accounting for the pain and expense encountered by those who survived it — we can see that it was experimental, whether the physician performing the operation regarded it this way or not. In virtually all therapies initially alleged to be curative and ultimately judged worthless, but never labeled as investigational, the public has been misled in this same manner.

34. This operation, developed by a Canadian surgeon named Arthur Vineberg, is done by cutting an artery free of the inside chest wall and tunneling it into the heart muscle, in the hope that blood will then flow through the artery into the ailing heart.

It is not unusual for research to escape the scrutiny of review boards by being conducted in the name of clinical practice. The physician has extensive prerogatives in this regard; unless the activity is designated as research or is under the purview of a research program, the physician can simply label his experiments unusual clinical practice. The famous case of the first artificial heart implantation was called a "therapeutic innovation" consistent with clinical practice and the surgeon's judgment of what was necessary for the patient, but analysis of the case leaves little doubt that the artificial heart was not even fit for human experimentation.[35] Unlike new drugs, new surgical procedures can be used without surveillance and without the label of experimentation. In private practice almost anything can be done under the rubric of therapy. Most medical practices are incomprehensible to patients and invisible to colleagues. Physicians may not consider their practices experiments, but from the perspective of the patient given unproven treatments, they are exactly that. We can only guess at how many patients are unwitting subjects of unrecognized experimentation.

REASONS FOR OVERTREATMENT

ECONOMIC INCENTIVES

> The test to which all methods of treatment are finally brought is whether they are lucrative to doctors or not.
>
> George Bernard Shaw,
> *The Doctor's Dilemma*

The physician is unique in being permitted to determine who needs his services. The jailer and the mortician also need to make a living, but we are careful not to let them decide who needs their services. Once sickness is pronounced, the physician is permitted, under the unwritten contract, to decide what his customers will buy. The usual rules of supply and demand do

35. Renee C. Fox and Judith P. Swazey, *The Courage to Fail*, pp. 149-211.

not apply, as the physician provides the service he orders. Unquestionably, the physician with a fee-for-service practice has a strong conflict of interest between his own financial gain and the best interests of his patients. Like the jeweler and the automobile salesman, he wants to sell as many of his products as he can and the most expensive ones when he can.

When a surgeon is faced with a choice between doing nothing, for which he collects a thirty-dollar consultation fee, and recommending surgery for which he would get three thousand dollars, is he not going to be influenced in the direction of surgery? Only a physician would dare suggest impartiality under the circumstances. The most honest person can not help being swayed by the enticement of money for the mere decision to do something—men and women simply do not resist such pressures—and when indications are marginal, or the type of treatment makes little difference in the long run, the decision will inevitably reflect the economic incentive.

Medical practices that are not profitable or that result in net financial loss have tended to become obsolete at space-age speed. The thorough physical examination and talking to the patient's family come to mind as low- or non-paying services that have almost disappeared. The doctor is in a position to obtain maximum economic return for his time, and the money in medicine is in procedures. The same physician who receives $30 for a forty-five-minute physical examination can get $120 for spending twenty minutes doing a nerve block.

The medical fee structure, supported by every form of insurance, makes a simple procedure several times as rewarding to the physician as a life-saving maneuver that does not involve the use of knife, tube or needle. Even limiting their charges to those allowed under Medicare, general physicians can effect a threefold increase in income by ordering a number of common laboratory procedures to be done in the office, while surgeons receive from three to seven times as much money for each hour spent in the operating room as for each hour of consultation in the office or at the bedside.[36] There is not a physician in private practice who does not recognize the need to have a "gimmick" by which he can increase his income almost at will. Endoscopy, bronchoscopy, electrocardiograms, all laboratory tests, needle biopsies, dialysis, X rays, catheterizations, scans and even skin testing provide means to amplify income—witness the flourishing activity in these procedures. There is a marked increase in the use of procedures when the physician profits from them compared to the rate of their use when he does not.[37] Although physicians may not make conscious decisions based on income, in practice the financial incentives are always in the direction of performing the procedure. These influences may be subtle, and not in the forefront of the physician's mind, but they are real and important.

Medical tests are expensive and profitable. It is common practice for pathologists to enter into contracts with hospitals under which they receive a percentage of the fees from all laboratory tests. Some pathologists make well over $250,000 a year from this source alone. The more modern the test and the more expensive the equipment needed to perform it, the greater the profit. When a hospital or clinic or private practitioner installs an expensive instrument, the number of tests done requiring that instrument will increase rapidly. Physicians know how many tests they must order to show a reasonable return on their investment, and they see to it that the blood analyzer, or the catheterization laboratory, or the open-heart surgery equipment is sufficiently used. Much of a specialist's practice is running laboratory tests, and like the surgeon who must consider the profit motive in recommending an operation, the laboratory-oriented physician supports his practice by ordering the tests he

36. Thomas P. Almy, "The Role of the Primary Physician in the Health-Care 'Industry,'" New England Journal of Medicine 304(1981):225.

37. Committee on Technology and Health Care, Medical Technology and the Health Care System (Washington, D.C.: National Academy of Sciences, 1979), p. 36; F. Sloan and B. Steinwald, "Determinants of Physicians' Fees," Journal of Business 47(1974):493-511.

performs. The overuse of medical tests in many instances is tantamount to plundering, but usually without the patient knowing it. The line between ordering tests for profit and for obtaining knowledge helpful in treating the patient becomes indistinct to doctors.

When doctors train to do the most expensive procedures and equip themselves with the most expensive instruments—then deny financial considerations in recommending surgery or an expensive test—we may well ask why they chose that means of practicing medicine. The key to financial profit in a medical practice is maneuvering the practice to maximal remuneration regardless of individual decisions. By specializing in a procedure and charging enough for each one done, the physician assures himself of sufficient wealth regardless of individual decisions. Once in position to profit, physicians trumpet a particular procedure through testimonials, uncontrolled studies and the public media. With sufficient demand for his services, the physician has the luxury of being ethical in individual decisions. The well-positioned physician who absolves himself of seeking personal gain by pointing to the help he has given his anguished patients or the symptomatic improvement he has provided through the use of marginally effective technology, forgets that in so doing he has chosen not to practice among the underprivileged whose medical needs are greater, or to work in preventive medicine, which is lower paying but produces greater benefits for everyone in the long run.

Although there are some physicians who are almost saintly in their abstention from profit-oriented practices, these are very few, and most doctors, who are as honest as any other professional group, indulge in unconscionable self-enrichment, however it may be rationalized as supporting the best medical system in the world. We may argue that it is the fault of the system and not of those mortals who operate within it, but those who profit have consistently and vigorously defended their financial practices against efforts to decrease the profiteering.

As a group, physicians enjoy more wealth and financial security than any other professionals. In contrast to their professed ideals and service orientation, physicians are extremely rich by any standard, and growing even richer. In 1939, physicians' earnings were less than twice as high as those of a broad category of other technical and professional people, but in 1975 their earnings were four times as high; their incomes have increased more than those in any other occupation, and have far outpaced inflation.[38] It can be argued that physicians are as deserving of wealth as other groups, such as businessmen or salesmen. But what is most insidious and unacceptable about the wealth of physicians is that in response to financial incentives they reshape medical practices from what they otherwise would be, violating the intent of the doctor-patient contract, harming patients, and defiling the profession.

THE NEED TO TREAT

Physicians, like other professionals, tend to do what they are trained to do, and they respond to clinical problems by doing what they are best able to do. A surgeon has called this tendency "function-lust"—the love of performing a function.[39] The accomplished surgeon who operates with speed and skill derives pleasure and satisfaction from his work, as any artisan or craftsman does. Function-lust tempts him to perform the function which he is capable of and enjoys doing whether it will benefit the patient or not. Furthermore, physicians who are trained in a particular technique feel a necessity to use the technique in order to maintain their skills and to fulfill their purpose. Just as a matador must fight bulls to remain what he is, surgeons or physicians with technical skills must use those skills or they lose their expertise and self-respect, as well as that of their colleagues and patients. A surgeon is not a surgeon

38. "Doctors' Fees—Free from the Law of Supply and Demand," *Science* 200(1978):30.
39. George Crile, *Surgery*, p. 132.

unless he is operating, and when a surgeon is faced with operating or referring a patient for nonsurgical therapy, he is likely to interpret the indications in favor of the knife.

The desire of the physician to do everything that he has been trained to do, regardless of relative benefit, has been called the "technological imperative."[40] The physician who is skilled in a certain procedure, or is trained to operate a highly complex diagnostic instrument, will invariably resort to the skill for all manner of clinical problems. The availability of the skill mandates its use, especially when indications are ambiguous and the physician has free rein in deciding to use it.

In practical terms, a patient is likely to receive the kind of treatment the healer he chooses to see is best at. A patient with a migraine headache will be treated with spinal manipulation by a chiropractor, with acupuncture by an acupuncturist, with herbs by a naturopath, with talk by a psychotherapist, and with X rays and drugs by a physician—and each will claim to have the correct approach. The result may be the same for all approaches, but the specific therapy is dictated by the training of the therapist.

Nowhere is this principle better demonstrated than in dealing with specialists. Theoretically, and probably in reality as well, the nonspecialist, or generalist (now commonly called family practitioner) is best suited by temperament and practice habits to direct a patient to the proper specialist if one is needed. If the patient refers himself to a specialist, he had better know what he is doing, for function-lust is never more compelling than for the specialist! The specialist by definition has advanced training in a narrow field of medicine, and spends most of his time performing his specialized function. Thus, the patient with midbody distress will get an X ray of the colon if he sees a gastroenterologist, a heart catheterization if he sees a cardiologist, and a series of tests of hormone function if he visits an endocrinologist.

40. Victor R. Fuchs, *Who Shall Live?*, p. 60.

The specialist epitomizes the extremes of physician behavior and practice, being the most biophysical and least holistic of physicians. If the average clinician treats the patient like a machine, ignoring all other factors influencing health, the specialist does not even consider the whole machine, but treats abnormalities localized to one part of the body, or even a part of an organ. Consequently, in this era of extreme specialization in medicine, in which a patient's medical care may be parcelled out among four or five specialists, the technological imperative of specialists using their technology and expertise results in a fragmented overapplication of medical treatments and procedures. The medical specialist is of inestimable value when his particular expertise is needed, but as one might, upon approaching a diamond specialist, expect to be sold a diamond, one should be equally prepared in approaching a medical specialist.

Since the overriding necessity of clinical practice is to do something, it is most unusual for a patient to escape from a visit to the doctor without experiencing some action, diagnostic or therapeutic. The assumption is that for every complaint, no matter how trivial, there may be a submerged disease which, if left undiscovered and untreated, will have disastrous consequences for the patient. For most physicians the dictum *primum non nocere* ("first, do no harm") is replaced by "first, do something."

Action is mandated by the basic therapeutic contract, which stipulates that the physician do what the patient is unable to do. Knowledge about what is happening is of less importance than action, and as a result, on both sides of the relationship there is a firm conviction that doing something is better than doing nothing; the patient does not pay to have nothing done. Rather than asking, "What is the utility and chance of success of this action?" the physician asks, "What action is possible that bears on the case?" Both patient and physician hope for beneficial action, but both prefer action with little chance of benefit to no action at all. The following case illustrates the desire, if not the absolute need, of the physician to act, however unlikely the benefit.

An elderly woman, very alert and active for her age, was brought to the hospital for replacement of an artificial pacemaker that was beginning to fail. The physician in charge had known the woman for many years, and was very fond of her and proud of his role in restoring her to an active life through the pacemaker treatment. While in the hospital, and apparently unrelated to her need for a pacemaker, the woman suffered a stroke that left her paralyzed on one side and unable to talk. The physician in charge was distraught, partly because of his real distress over the woman's misfortune, but also because of his inability to do anything to help. The usual treatment at that time, blood-thinners, was prohibited by the consulting neurologist who wanted to wait in order to make sure that the stroke was not the kind made worse by blood-thinners. After about thirty-six hours, during which time the physician in charge repeatedly expressed his frustration at not being able to act, the neurologist gave approval for using blood-thinners, but cautioned that they were unlikely to be of help, and could still possibly cause harm. The physician in charge immediately began treatment with blood-thinners, remarking, "Thank God! Now we can do something."

The physician perceives the need for effective therapy, and translates it into a need for action, of any type, but the need to help gets confused with benefit of the action. As a consequence, when a patient takes a turn for the worse, the need to act propels the physician to use therapies of marginal or dubious benefit. As the patient's outlook worsens, the physician begins to justify any action, ironically placing the patient at greater risk. Futhermore, in a split decision over whether a particular treatment or test is indicated, activity usually wins the moment. If one physician thinks a test should be done and another thinks it shouldn't be done, the proponent almost always will prevail partly because the dissenter hesitates to block anything with a remote chance of helping. It is not uncommon for one strong advocate of a medical act to prevail over four or five colleagues who dissent.

When the physician learns to react to a crisis with heroic action, it is inevitable that he will begin to see all clinical problems in a crisis perspective. All clinical problems become potential emergencies, and no line is drawn between the situation where the emergency is real and there is little to lose from action, and pseudo- or potential emergencies in which there is little to be lost from inaction until more information can be acquired. In the early 1970s patients with coronary artery disease who had chest pain while resting were pronounced emergencies, and were sent for open-heart surgery. After thousands of patients had emergency operations, evidence accumulated showing that the situation did not represent an emergency and that such surgery was not of benefit.

The need to do something is so great that physicians usually will act even when success seems unlikely, as shown in the following account:

An 86-year-old man was brought to the hospital because of heart failure (evidenced by shortness of breath). All known drugs had been used, and there was no surgically correctable abnormality. One finding, however, was atrial fibrillation, a condition causing an irregular and slightly inefficient heartbeat, which perhaps contributed to the patient's breathing difficulty. A review of the evidence pointed to a statistical likelihood of success in correcting the abnormality by electrical shock (drugs had not worked) but likelihood of failure in maintaining the correction for more than a few days, and a considerable risk of complication in a man of this age. Overall, the predicted outcome from doing the procedure was greater chance of harm than benefit. When asked for an opinion as to what to do with this evidence in hand, three of four physicians responded in favor of using the electrical shock treatment. When asked why, in the face of near-certain failure and possible harm, one of the physicians replied, "But there is no other option." The only option was doing nothing. Doing something clearly was more important than being guided by the probable benefit or harm of the act.

The ultimate extension of doing something is doing everything possible. When the clinical situation deteriorates, the pressure to do everyting possible far outweighs any cool analysis of the relative potential benefits and harm of the acts. If the family of the sick person knows of an applicable diagnostic test or therapy, they will push for it without inquiring further. They make the fallacious assumption, often shared by the physician, that any available treatments would not exist if they were not of benefit. The physician practicing alone is able to resist such entreaties from the family if he is resolute in his opinion and can marshal convincing evidence against the proposed action, but when decisions are observed by colleagues, peer pressure to act can be as forceful as that from the family or the patient.

The physician who holds out against what he believes is unnecessary or unhelpful action will usually succumb to pressure to act when death appears imminent, if only to remove doubt about whether the proposed action would have worked. The physician, as well as the patient's family, who feel responsibility for management of their loved one's illness, can always at the end say, "At least we tried," or "We gave it our best." The patient, who usually has no say in his own management, is subjected to treatment whose benefit is not probable but is only remotely possible. In the despair of impending disaster, those close to the patient have the natural but irrational urge to stop at nothing, to grasp every straw, to reach back for the ultimate superstitious act of believing in the omnipotence of the physician.

I seldom have seen a physician able to resist doing everything possible in a desperate situation. It is the ultimate expression of the healer who in the name of compassion and fulfillment of the basic contract performs an act predictably of no benefit and most likely to increase suffering. That the act is seen by the credulous family as a heroic effort to save their loved one speaks to the need of the family for such belief. I suspect that the only participant in the drama able to take full measure of the act, the patient, is unable to respond effectively and must exit this world disillusioned but with fuller comprehension of the healer.

The physician believes that doing everything possible is consistent with ethical practice. If the patient dies or suffers excessively, the physician feels defenseless if he has not done everything possible. The standard of conduct is doing everything another physician might have done under similar circumstances; from a professional perspective, conduct is more important than results. Results are seen as not always within the physician's control. Things can go wrong at any time: Every treatment has its risks as a matter of chance. But conduct is under control of the doctor, and proper conduct under the unwritten doctor-patient contract, as well as the professional code, is to do everything possible. The professional need to treat is a great unrecognized cause of iatrogenic harm.

In summary, we do not know how much avoidable iatrogenic harm occurs because we have no standards for what is necessary or appropriate practice. All surgery poses a risk, and in the best hands some appropriate surgery will fail or result in harm. Although not negligible, harm from appropriate therapy is an acceptable risk; harm from inappropriate practices is not acceptable. Physicians, economists and others, looking at the medical field as professionals, estimate that one-half to three-quarters of all therapy is unnecessary. Those who purchase the product, the consumers, presumably accept as necessary whatever the doctor prescribes, else they wouldn't take it. But are they well-informed consumers, or do they automatically assume that the doctor knows best and is serving their interests, as people have believed throughout most of history?

To err may be human, but "human error" implies a chance mistake not likely to be repeated. Iatrogenic harm occasionally represents pardonable human error, but for the most part, it is born of professional and economic incentives and of disregard for the well-being of patients. The errors that result in iatrogenic harm are systematic, and they are avoidable.

The question remains: Does overall benefit exceed overall harm of medical practices? When patients with curable diseases are treated, there is a real and valuable net positive gain. The vast area of harm is in medical intervention for those who don't need it or intervention of the kind for which there is no evidence of benefit. Iatrogenesis ensues from application of curing when caring is needed. Harm is the inevitable side effect of the emphasis on physician-dominated encounter medicine rather than medicine that strengthens the primary determinants of health—environment, nutrition and behavior.

CHAPTER EIGHT

The Fundamental Deception of Medicine

"Don't you think men overrate the necessity for humoring every-body's nonsense till they get despised by the very fools they humour?" said [Dr.] Lydgate . . . . "The shortest way is to make your value felt so that people must put up with you whether you flatter them or not."

"With all my heart," responded Mr. Farebrother. "But then you must be sure of having the value, and you must keep yourself independent. Very few men can do that. Either you slip out of service altogether and become good for nothing or you wear the harness and draw a good deal where your yoke-fellows pull you."

George Eliot,
Middlemarch

A lie is only useful as a medicine to men. The use of such medicines should be confined to physicians.

Plato,
The Republic

T HE FUNDAMENTAL deception of medicine, the notion that doctors have special healing powers, endures because society demands it and the medical profession insti-tutionalizes it. It arises from the basic doctor-patient contract, which defines the patient as dependent and the doctor as om-nipotent and which regulates almost all medical practices, whether the healing system be scientific medicine, acupuncture, homeopathy or voodoo.

THE DECEPTION OF THE HEALER

Most people would argue that they don't see their physicians as having supernatural powers, that they are surely sophisticated enough not to look upon their doctors as priests. But common practice belies the denial. Although people generally do not revere their physicians when they are well, when they are sick, they regress to the most irrational dependency. How often have you heard someone say, "Doctor, whatever you say, I'll do"? Does a person have such blind faith in his plumber or a taxi driver? Would he so readily let someone do whatever he wanted to his automobile? Have you ever really questioned your doctor, to his face? Such faith in the doctor is hard to shake not only because the individual lacks the means of assessing the doctor's practice, but precisely because he does not want to know exactly what the doctor is capable of. The alternative to faith in the doctor is the reality of being in the hands of a fallible human being who has limited power to act against diseases.

The healer is as easily seduced into believing in his special powers as his patients are, as we saw in the case of Quesalid. The very first healer who assumed the supernatural powers willed upon him by a desperate patient was the first to fall in with this deception, and the medical profession has yet to renounce him or give up the inherited assumption of superiority in curing. Nurtured by clinical success and the acclaim of patients, the deception of the healer has been passed down from teacher to student for thousands of years. That those who followed in this tradition accepted it as part of their training makes them no less culpable than their superstitious forebears; on the contrary, the advent of science in medicine ought surely to have caused this idea to be questioned and rejected at least a hundred years ago. Instead, the tremendous power of the profession and the energy and resources of its members are marshaled to support the belief.

Physicians will no doubt protest this allegation. But again, practice speaks louder than words. The physician may not claim to have special powers, but he behaves as if he had them when he disdains scientific evidence in favor of his own hunches, when he excludes patients from participating in decisions about their own care, and when he defends his right to exercise these prerogatives—when, in short, he behaves like an Aesculapian priest.

The Aesculapian priests may have believed their own claims, but if they did, they deceived themselves as well as their patients who arose from the therapeutic ritual attributing their sense of well-being to the supernatural powers of the priests. Patients today undergo the same sort of ceremony when they have coronary bypass surgery. They spend several days at the temple (hospital) prior to the ultimate healing act. During this time, they are given much encouragement; they are told of how they will be cured;[1] they are prepared with special diets and purgings; they read pamphlets—a modern version of votive tablets—describing the cure; and they receive news of the cure from patients who have preceded them. On the night before the cure they are taken to the scene of the ceremony, the method of the cure is described to them, and they are shown where they will awaken afterwards. There are very few patients who are not convinced that they will be cured by the eve of their bypass operation. When it is time for the operation, they are taken to the inner chamber of the temple and put to sleep. They awaken healed. The emotional response to the preparation for the operation, and the intense belief that it will cure them are undoubtedly as effective as the rituals of the Aesculapian priests were. When a patient responds to the ritual, today as three thousand years ago, and is told that the specific act—the operation— caused the healing, he is deceived, for the healing power of this experience resides in the patient's mind.

If healing is due not so much to the drugs and operations we use as to the authority with which we use them, is perpetuating the myth not justified? Wouldn't it be callous and emotionally devastating to deprive patients of beliefs that we can see ease their minds and in fact stimulate natural healing?

1. In this passage I use *cure* not to mean a specific cure as I defined it in Chapter 3, but to mean a general healing, thought of as a "cure" by the patients who undergo this operation.

Think of the man who has severe viral pneumonia, the kind that is not cured by antibiotics. The physician knows the virus won't respond to antibiotics, but prescribes them anyway, rationalizing that there may be a hidden bacterial component to the disease that will be cured, and that the drug will "do no harm." The patient is put in the hospital where he is given the drug with the usual assurance of its effectiveness, and he dutifully recovers. The patient thinks his recovery was due to the specific healing properties of the drug. In this case, was the treatment justified or not?

Unquestionably the treatment worked: The patient's belief in the benefit of the drug gave him the hope and encouragement necessary to mobilize his own natural defenses, which are extremely important to any successful therapy. But was the deception necessary? Weren't there alternative means of offering emotional support? Clearly there were. The really good doctor, without practicing any deception at all, could have told the patient with warmth and interest that although antibiotics would be of no benefit, the patient's own defenses and the support of nursing care would help him recover, and that all the resources of modern medicine were on standby for use if and when they would be helpful. In the end, the patient's trust in the doctor would be just as great, if not greater, but it would be a trust in the physician's ability to care and to give sound expert advice, not a blind faith in a healer or a drug. In addition, the patient would not have received a potentially harmful drug, but would have come to understand the power of his own natural healing abilities.

The difference between the Aesculapian priests and modern physicians is that today's doctors have access to genuinely curative therapies. Given these cures, it is no longer necessary to rely on a myth that may have been of value when faith and hope were the only remedies available to the ill person. When curative technologies are not enough, hope and natural healing powers can still be mobilized by the love and support of people who care. As Norman Cousins, who achieved natural healing, so aptly put it, the heaviest artillery against illness is the will to live.[2]

Most people think of healing as being "enshrouded in mystery," but this is illusion, for there is no mystery. The heart surgeon, doing intricate surgery with the most sophisticated technological assistance, doesn't have any special skills or knowledge that the average person couldn't learn with training. Laboratory technicians who do the same operations on animals—and veterinarians, for that matter—are denied the same status as the heart surgeon, even though their work is nearly identical to his. The curative powers of Western medicine lie not in the individual physician, but in the body of scientific knowledge that is available to all of us. There are differences among physicians, to be sure: Some have better technical skills than others, and some are better than others at mobilizing a patient's natural healing powers. But when the modern physician cures by using an antibiotic or an operation, he deceives the patient and himself by allowing the notion that his role was indispensable. The deception of the healer allows every physician to become—in greater or lesser measure—a Quesalid.

THE DECEPTION OF AUTHORITY

The exaggerated authority and power of doctors may be forced on them to satisfy a public demand for "healers" whose special powers will protect us against the frightening irrationality of disease. But once the physician assumes the authority, he begins to resist scientific, impartial assessment of his remedies because such evaluation questions his judgment, and he regards trust in his judgment as essential to his ability to heal. In defense of his remedies, the physician often uses some of the same practices as quacks, e.g., simulating science in the application of therapies; using post hoc, ergo propter hoc reasoning to associate therapies

2. Norman Cousins, Anatomy of an Illness.

with apparent cures; remembering cures and forgetting failures; claiming credit for the placebo effect of persuasion and suggestion in therapy; using testimonials as the primary source of evidence of benefit of therapies; treating people who have no symptoms but who "may have underlying disease"; and rejecting critical scrutiny—testing—and insisting upon secrecy in evaluation of practices (only physicians are allowed to judge physicians).

Physicians argue that scrutiny of practices within the medical establishment does occur, marking a major difference from the practices of quacks and healers. This contention is based first on confusing self-serving tests of their own practices with scientific scrutiny (as I shall discuss in more detail in the next section). Second, physicians hold the mistaken belief that testing of the operational reliability of a practice (i.e., the effectiveness of an antibiotic to kill bacteria, or the technical success of an operation) is the same as testing for the benefit of the practice.

Does it matter that penicillin has been scientifically proved to kill bacteria if the clinician uses it to treat the common cold, which is not caused by bacteria? Is that not as superstitious as the quack's using snake oil to treat arthritis? Machines that produce radiation are the product of brilliant scientific discoveries, but was the harmful use of irradiation to shrink thymus glands any less reprehensible than the use of linament for the treatment of tuberculosis?

A patient can easily distinguish between the credentials of a physician and a quack by noting place of practice, diplomas and other professional trappings, but the reckless and untested claims of physicians make it difficult for the public to differentiate between the practices of physicians and quacks. Consider, for instance, the controversial drug laetrile. Why do most physicians oppose it? Because it is scientifically unproven? That is the usual answer, but what evidence do we have that most of the anticancer drugs and procedures that have been used over the last twenty years are beneficial to patients (quite aside from their effects on mice)? Physicians are inconsistent when they insist on rigorous confirmation of the benefit of therapies originating from other belief systems, but strenuously resist scientific evaluations of the therapies they themselves apply and believe in.

A physician who denounced laetrile as worthless insisted that coronary bypass surgery makes patients better, "because the patients tell you they are better." But there never has been a scientific study showing that symptom relief following coronary bypass surgery is due to anatomic changes, and there is a great deal of evidence that the operation has a powerful placebo effect. Laetrile patients also claim that they are better. Is this method of evaluation for one treatment any more or less valid than it is for the other? The public, discerning no difference, accepts both claims as valid. The medical profession condemns the public for its consistency, believing that professional pronouncement ought to be sufficient evidence of what is good therapy and what is not. But, historically, the medical profession has conditioned the public to accept therapies without scientific evidence of safety or benefit, so when patients evaluate laetrile on the basis of testimonials, they are doing exactly what the medical profession has taught them to do for the last four thousand years.

DECEPTIVE CLINICAL PRACTICES

There is probably no area in which deception is more widespread in medicine than in the accumulation and dissemination of clinical knowledge. As we have seen, most of the "knowledge" on which therapy has been based has been incorrect, but, at every stage in the history of medicine, the knowledge of contemporary doctors was considered authoritative. Discarded practices might be disdained as superstition or inaccuracy, but current practices always have been believed to be true and accurate. Galen's deception was not in having inaccurate or incomplete information—a problem that will always be with us—but in so heartily accepting without question existing beliefs, and thereby promulgating the untruths of his day. Truth in medicine is hard to come by, and there are very few areas of medical practice where the whole truth is readily accessible. Refusal to acknowledge lack of information about important medical problems constitutes deception.

Further deception about medical knowledge takes two forms. The first, relatively uncommon, is deliberate lying. Physicians may lie about what tests show, what was actually done to a patient, or the real results of a therapy. They may fake findings in medical investigations in order to gain approval for a specific procedure or therapy.[3] This kind of deception is not unique to medicine. It occurs in any endeavor where personal recognition and profit are at stake. Although it is more common in medicine than the public wishes to believe, it is not a systematic flaw that might be eliminated by changing professional norms, since the profession already condemns it.

A second type of deception is systematic and grows out of the notion of the special powers of healers. This is the belief that the physician's own clinical judgment is superior to scientific knowledge derived from carefully controlled studies and investigations. This deception is perpetuated by accepted methods of assessing medical practices.

The assessment of therapy by those who provide it is one of the most astonishing inconsistences in Western society. In no other sphere of public life is the producer of a service or product pronounced the sole evaluator and protected as such by the law, with no real attempt by those who receive the service to make a comprehensive assessment of it. This is comparable to politicians being the sole judges of their actions, or automobile dealers being the sole appraisers of the vehicles they sell.

Most evaluation of therapy has nothing to do with the exper-

3. C. Holden, "FDA Tells Senators of Doctors Who Fake Data in Clinical Drug Trials," *Science* 206(1979):432; Renee C. Fox and Judith P. Swazey, *The Courage to Fail*, p. 159; "Cancer Research Data Falsified; Boston Project Collapses," *Boston Sunday Globe*, June 29, 1980, p. 1.

tise needed to administer it, but rather requires careful rec-
ordkeeping, unbiased interviewing, and a knowledge of statistics, skills in which most physicians are notably deficient.
Physicians believe that only physicians are capable of judging
other physicians and their acts, and that only a specialist is
capable of judging another specialist. As a consequence, all of
those who might be able to give an impartial assessment within
the profession are excluded, and of course scrutiny from outside
the profession is absolutely prohibited.

Nonmedical businesses understand perfectly well that independent evaluation of techniques or products is essential to
obtain a reasonably accurate assessment of their quality and
value, and so they commonly employ independent agencies to
test new products and designs, agencies who have no stake in
the soundness of the practice or product, but whose reputation
depends on accurate testing and reporting. But the physician
who applies a new cancer therapy is the same person who
pronounces it a success, and both his colleagues and his patients
believe him because we are all raised to do so without question.
The physician has the right to argue, to give evidence and even
to plead for the practice in question, but he should not have the
right to try his own case. If the goal were to serve the best
interests of the public, without consideration for professional
gain, physicians would seek unbiased assessment of their
practices.

Trickery and deception used to induce patients to accept a
particular therapy or diagnostic test is common in clinical practice. The physician who believes that something is beneficial for
the patient does not hesitate to use deceptive means to persuade
the unwilling patient that it must be done. Telling the patient
that he will probably die without an operation is an effective
technique, but usually it is a blatant lie. At best a physician can
give odds about the probability of survival with the treatment
and the probability of survival without it, but he can never be
sure of the outcome for any given patient. Even when physicians

believe what they tell patients, if they make unvalidated claims, their deception is no less than that of the psychic surgeon, who also believes in his therapy. For years physicians told patients that the Vineberg operation was necessary to save their lives, but there is to date not a shred of scientific evidence that the operation prolonged life.

In clinical practice, deception sometimes becomes necessary to sustain the effect of prior deception. A difficult clinical problem arose in the case of a man who had coronary artery surgery for relief of chest pain. Before the operation the man was told that the chance of relieving his pain was almost certain, and that his chances of living longer also would be greatly improved. After the operation, the patient reported no pain and said he felt "like a new man" who had been "rescued from death." Unfortunately, on a routine re-examination six months later, X rays showed closure of all the bypass grafts, meaning that the operation was a total failure.[4] Many physicians would have told the patient of this finding, but because the man was feeling so well, and because the doctor in charge feared undoing the therapeutic effect of the operation, he chose to withhold the information from the patient, who continued relatively pain-free and happy and attributed his recovery to the operation.

The rationale for this deception, not uncommon in medicine, was that full disclosure of the findings would have been injurious to the patient, and that it was in the best interests of the patient not to receive information that would undermine the therapeutic result or the doctors. It is very much like the "white lies" that most of us tell in our daily lives to "protect the other person."

But in matters involving health professionals and members of the public, it is essential to look at the problem from a different perspective. What is the difference between this doctor and the

4. The majority of patients who have unsuccessful coronary artery surgery report relief of pain and improved lifestyle. Fortunately, only about one in twenty patients has a totally unsuccessful operation, although about one in four operations is not totally successful in the technical sense.

quack who deceives with psychic surgery? In both instances the healer is willing to use deception to attain the therapeutic goal.

Is the man who had unsuccessful coronary artery surgery better off not knowing it? As long as successful therapy depends on *belief* in a healer or a drug or an operation, then maintenance of the belief, by any means, becomes more important than the actual therapy. The patient with the unsuccessful operation got short-term protection, but someday he may find out what really happened, and if he does, the blow will be all the more cruel, for the psychological support necessary to sustain the therapy will then be irrevocably withdrawn. Furthermore, he will lose faith not only in the physicians who deceived him, but likely in the entire medical establishment, and be discouraged from seeking the real benefits of modern medicine.

THE PLACEBO DECEPTION

The essence of deception in medicine is the placebo, an ineffective but presumably harmless agent the patient is given thinking that he is receiving a curative therapy. Every doctor knows that if a placebo merely convinces a patient of the therapist's interest in and attempt to do something for him, it will produce a profound relief of symptoms. Any potion of sugar-water will make a patient feel better if he believes the potion is curative.

A noted contemporary medical economist wrote, without condoning the practice, "The use of placebos undoubtedly adds to the public's expenditures for drugs, but it is not clear whether there is any less expensive way of dealing with the cases for which they are typically prescribed."[5] In other words, the placebo deception may be economically justified. Even Plato recognized the use of placebos, and understood their effect. In *The Republic* he wrote, "A lie is only useful as a medicine to men. The use of such medicines should be confined to physicians." But if the true extent and cost of the deception were

5. Victor R. Fuchs, *Who Shall Live?*, p. 125.

known, I believe reasonable men would not accept placebos either as an economic expedient or as "a medicine to men."

The placebo is sometimes given knowingly, even cavalierly. The doctor will prescribe a sugar pill or an injection of salt water and tell the patient that the "medicine" will make him well. This leads to such things as asking for antibiotics for every cold, seeking useless operations for imagined maladies, and a general feeling of inability to cope without the assistance of a physician. Worse yet, if the deception is discovered, the patient loses trust in all physicians. Patients who realize they have been duped often engage in counterplacebo activity, feigning the taking of drugs. Then the physician is duped, for he may come to believe in the benefit of a drug that is not even being taken. Some patients feel no remorse in deceiving their physicians, and physicians suspect almost all patients of not following their directions. The result can become a game of deception and counterdeception that no one wins.

Many physicians refuse to deliberately administer a placebo because of the guile involved. According to hospital corridor ethics, it is acceptable to give a placebo knowingly "for the patient's good," but only when there is no reasonable alternative. As a naked act, it is a slightly disreputable practice within the profession.

The unrecognized placebo, or the partially recognized placebo, is more common. If the physician has moral qualms about using a pure placebo, he can avoid guilt by using a therapy that has some benefit, or that he thinks may have. Some clinicians openly advocate the use of partially effective treatments—for example, tranquilizers—as placebos, arguing that the deception is minimized by the existence of at least a possibility of real benefit. The danger is in the escalation from harmless sugar capsules to partially effective drugs to dangerous therapies such as toxic drugs or surgery. Searching for more effective means of bringing about healing, the physician reaches for ever more powerful therapies. In the progression from the inert placebo consciously given to the active procedure thought to have a profound physical effect, the physician fills his therapeutic arsenal with unrecognized placebos, and becomes unable to differentiate between the truly curative and the placebo components coexisting in most therapies. He confuses the physical or chemical effect of the treatment with the patient's response to it. He fails to recognize that even the patient who has undergone open-heart surgery will respond not only to the physiologic effects of the operation, but also to the expectation that it will make him well.

Unfortunately, there is no final solution to the problem of placebos. Doctors will very likely always use them in some form. Proper testing to find what portion of recovery is due to the placebo effect could eliminate therapies which are mostly or partially placebos—such as tranquilizers, hormone shots and unnecessary operations—and substitute treatments that are truly curative, with less risk and expense to the public, and without deception.

DECEPTION IN DISABILITY

In return for complete authority in handling diseases, the doctor-patient contract stipulates the willingness of the physician to acknowledge and sometimes support the patient's perception of his problems. The distinction between disease and illness is important: The physician alone determines the presence of disease, but the patient alone can express how the problem affects him—that is, his illness. Acquiescence in this part of the contract invites deception on both sides. The patient can achieve personal gain by claiming unreal disability and abusing the social welfare system if he can get a doctor to certify that he is sick. Requests for sick leave, retirement, disability benefits and the like, supported by exaggerated or distorted diagnoses, require the collusion of the physician. Most physicians go along with this deception most of the time, either reasoning that everyone else does it and this patient is as deserving of a handout as the next person, or simply not wishing to upset the doctor-patient relationship. Although this bothers many physicians, it is nearly universal in medical practice, and is commonplace in disability cases and on both sides of medical malpractice suits. Because the doctor does not allow questioning of his pronouncements, he must acquiesce in claims over which the patient is granted authority by the contract. In this way each party supports the deceptions of the other.

DECEPTION IN RESEARCH AND INVESTIGATION

Many patients are not informed of the investigational nature of the procedures being performed upon them, despite a growing public awareness of their need to know when treatment is experimental. Deceptive investigational practices in medicine were unchecked until the last couple of decades, and even though there are now protective government regulations, experimental abuses of subjects through the use of deceptive techniques are widely reported in both the medical and the social sciences.[6]

Sometimes, of course, the nature of the research requires withholding information from the subject. The identity of a drug, for example, might be withheld in order to eliminate psychological effects. If a subject willingly agrees to enter an investigation in which he will not know whether the capsule he receives contains sugar or an active drug, and if he is able to opt out of the experiment should he desire, he is not deceived by the practice. He should, however, have access to full details of the treatment on request, and should be told the relative benefits and risks of the experiment. When experimentation is actually labeled as such, the rights of patients are now fairly well protected by review boards of the institutions conducting the research. But there ought to be more public participation on the

6. "Cancer Research Data Falsified"; Sissela Bok, *Lying*, pp. 193-95.

review boards to insure that the interests of the experimental subjects are fully represented.

The problem is that much medical investigation is not labeled as research. All new therapies are investigational, and when a physician uses one, he deceives his patient if he doesn't reveal that it is experimental. Coronary bypass surgery was clearly an investigational therapy for many years and yet patients were not told of its true status. For five years or more after the operation became common, doctors had very little understanding of which patients would benefit from it and which ones were likely to die from it. During this period the average patient had as good a chance of living without the operation as with it, but from the very first operation, it was not even thought of as investigational by the profession. We need to recognize that undisclosed experimental therapy arises from professional attitudes of superiority and paternalism, and that it will end only when those attitudes change.

THE DECEPTION OF MEDICAL ETHICS

Medical ethics, as the phrase is used by the profession, is deceptive because it is misleading. It means medical etiquette and does not address the interaction between doctor and patient or the effects of medical intervention on a patient. Since the patient is the vulnerable one in the doctor-patient relationship, true medical ethics should center on him—should deal with his rights, feelings and well-being, and the human values that are at stake in medical decision-making.[7]

Unfortunately, medical ethics as seen from the physician's perspective and promulgated in professional codes exist to enforce the concept of exclusivity and special status and the belief

7. The codes of Nuremberg, Geneva and Helsinki were written from the perspective of the patient, as have been other statements of patients' legal rights (see George J. Annas, *The Rights of Hospital Patients: An American Civil Liberties Union Handbook*), but none of these originated as professional guidelines. They were written largely by nonmedical individuals and groups.

that only doctors are qualified to make ethical decisions in the practice of medicine, a belief that allows physicians to consider themselves answerable only to colleagues in their particular field. This position is elitist at best, and confuses professional expertise with other qualities that are possessed by the laity as well as by physicians. To claim sole ability to make ethical judgments affecting the welfare of other people is an astonishing expression of arrogance and disregard for those whom physicians purport to serve.

The medical professional codes are attempts to regulate professional conduct for the benefit of the profession, which may be appropriate and essential for organizational stability and efficiency. But they fail to address the obligation of physicians to be accountable to their clients, to subordinate professional and personal incentives when they are in conflict with patients' needs, and to avoid deception in any form in medical practice. Reliance on existing codes of ethics gives both physicians and patients a false sense that the real ethical questions have been dealt with, when in truth they have scarcely even been acknowledged.

There is an awareness among many physicians of the need for patient-centered ethical thinking, and the physician's *personal* code of ethics, as distinct from his professional codes, generally favors the patient. But the influences of professional norms and practices overpower and often push aside personal ethics. Until the medical profession and the public can agree upon and institutionalize a true code of ethics that is subject to popular scrutiny and accepted by physicians, we deceive ourselves by believing that medical ethics are adequate to protect the rights and meet the needs of patients.

THE RISKS OF DECEPTION

As we have seen, deception in clinical medicine is not random and individual; it is part of accepted professional practice. Medical students learn subtle deceptions by example, by observing their teachers and senior colleagues. From using evasive or incomprehensible language to exclude the patient from communication among professionals at the bedside, to conscious lying about the purpose or result of a test, deception of the patient is systematically if unconsciously taught to the medical student from the beginning of his clinical experience, all in support of the notion of the healer.

We must count the cost of this deception and ask whether this is what we want from our medical schools and from the profession in which we place so much trust. There are grave physical risks to the patient who gets ineffective, harmful or unnecessary therapy. A concomitant risk is the patient's loss of control over decisions concerning his own health. By manipulating information or using coercive techniques, the physician strips the patient of his right to self-determination and personal responsibility, so that the patient is cheated of nothing less than his right to participate in decisions that may make the difference between life and death.

Deception carries risks for physicians, too. The deceptive notion of the healer forces the doctor to treat even when treatment is inappropriate, in order to maintain his image as healer. It prevents him from being truly holistic by compelling him to stay within the bounds of his particular belief system. Thus, the physician may treat only biophysically, the chiropractor must always manipulate the skeleton and the psychotherapist must stick to a particular theory. To fulfill his role, the physician must often compromise himself. In most cases he feels that he cannot tell a patient that no curative therapy is necessary. To do so would invite financial disaster, for the average doctor knows that if he is scrupulously honest in admitting that he often has nothing of curative value to offer, he will soon find himself with no patients, for the naked truth has no appeal to the patient programed to seek curative therapy as a substitute for caring. The subservience of the clinician to the demands of the public often reaches incredible heights. The incessant demand for tranquilizers, sick leave or disability benefits, drugs or operations, hospitalization to avoid expenses or to get away from problems at home are enough to make the physician with a conscience seriously contemplate a career in research.

Ultimately, the physician and the medical profession are at risk of being discredited because of deceptive practices. Much of the present movement away from conventional medicine to alternative methods can be traced directly to public disillusionment with deceptive professional claims. In the confusion, there is a dissillusionment with science itself that prevents careful investigation of the claims of alternative practitioners and throws medicine back into a prescientific morass of superstition and fads. If the medical profession had established a policy of vigorous opposition to unvalidated and deceptive claims, more people would go to doctors and be more willing to refrain from their own countercoercions. If most medical therapies had not been built on deceptive practices, the quacks and faith healers who flourish could not as easily fool people with the same techniques.

The systematic incorporation of deceptive methods, largely unrecognized by the profession, annuls the clause in the basic contract in which the physician agrees to act in the best interests of the patient, and degrades the practice of medicine.

CHAPTER NINE

The Need for Public Involvement in Medicine

All scientific endeavor is a social phenomenon . . . . After all, the social, national, country-wide implications of medicine are as old as this country . . . . I am not competent to have any views on the very difficult problem of the relations between the medical profession and society. But the notion that it is just an individual affair between a patient and a doctor seems to me totally discredited by all we know.

> Felix Frankfurter,
> Justice of the U.S. Supreme Court

In the main, then, the doctor learns that if he gets ahead of the superstitions of his patients he is a ruined man; and the result is that he instinctively takes care not to get ahead of them. That is why all the changes come from the laity.

> George Bernard Shaw,
> *The Doctor's Dilemma*

THE EXTRAORDINARY control physicians exercise over individual patients under the basic contract, insofar as it conforms to the standards of the medical profession, is virtually outside the jurisdiction of the state. With the contract as its source of power, the medical profession extends its authority over the entire public in three ways: (1) it controls the quality and availability of conventional health care services; (2) it determines the cost of health care and the allocation of public medical funds; and (3) by defining some social and moral issues as medical problems, it preempts society's right to decide how these problems will be viewed and dealt with.

The abuse of power in medicine is sanctioned by society, accepted by the public, and instilled into the behavior of medical students. The profession has become so independent of its clients and immune to outside influences that it is a formidable deterrent to changes that would be in the public interest. An eminent physician has written:

> The medical establishment is not primarily engaged in the disinterested pursuit of knowledge and the translation of that knowledge into medical practice; rather in significant part it is engaged in special interest advocacy, pursuing and preserving social power. . . . Professionalism has perpetuated prevailing practices, deflected criticism, and insulated the profession from alternative views and social relations that would illuminate and improve health care.[1]

CONTROL OF MEDICAL SERVICES

To the casual observer it may seem that modern medicine is mutually beneficial to patient and doctor. A great number and variety of services are available, doctors have full employment, and the government and private insurance companies foot most of the bill. But closer examination reveals that the medical profession has control over health matters that ought to be under public jurisdiction.

Doctors determine what services are available and when, who is eligible for them, where doctors' offices and hospitals are located, how many specialists and generalists practice medicine, the quality of health services (which practices are acceptable and which are not), and the cost of health care. The few attempts by the government to intervene in health care have been concerned only with funding—Medicare in the United States and national health insurance plans in other countries. U.S. Public Law 92-603, enacted in 1973 to establish mandatory cost and quality controls through Professional Standard Review Organizations, does not seek to review the *benefit* of professional practices but to guarantee conformity to standards set by the profession. Government insurance plans make sure that

1. H.R. Holman, "The 'Excellence' Deception in Medicine," *Hospital Practice* 11(1976):11.

people can afford medical services but do not seek to regulate the services themselves — to make sure that they are beneficial instead of harmful. Government money has the effect of increasing the domination of physicians by supporting their practices and therefore their power and autonomy.

With the exception of China and Cuba today, medical practice never has been regulated from outside. Even Hitler could not control his physicians, as seen from the report of Dr. Karl Gebhardt, who was called in to treat Reinhard Heydrich, the Chief of the Security Service and Deputy Protector of Bohemia and Moravia, who had been shot:

> In the extraordinary excitement and nervous tension which prevailed and was not diminished by daily personal telephone calls from Hitler and Himmler in person, asking for information, very many suggestions were naturally made . . . . I did not hesitate to take personal responsibility and state my own view, as to which I had no doubts. I consider that if anything endangers a patient it is nervous tension at the bedside and the appearance of too many doctors. I refused, in reply to direct demands, to call in any other doctor, not even Morell (Hitler's personal physician) or Sauerbruch. Heydrick died in fourteen days.[2]

The barefoot doctors in China were not recruited only to provide doctors where none had existed before; they were rather a political creation to wrest power away from the profession and give it to other political groups.[3] The new Communist government, unable to change the profession to meet what it perceived as community needs, could eliminate the power of the profession in controlling medical practices and making medical policy only by taking it away from physicians beholden to the profession, and giving it to health workers responsible to community governments. Defining illness and determining who was sick became no longer the sole province of the physician reacting to professional norms, but became the business of the community

2. M. Siegler and H. Osmond, "Aesculapian Authority," *Hastings Center Studies* 1(1973):41.

3. S.B. Rifkin, "Politics of Barefoot Medicine," *Lancet* 1(1978):34.

or the political party. Allocation of resources was no longer dictated by personal interests and financial motives of physicians, but by the perceived needs of the community.

According to one analyst, there are few, if any, other countries where the migration of health professionals from poorer to wealthier communities has been reversed and where low-cost, primary-care services appear to be available six days a week—and often on evenings and holidays—in places easily accessible to those who need the care.[4] This account is not intended as either an endorsement or an indictment of the Chinese system, but as a clear-cut example of the political nature of medicine, about which I shall say a good deal more later.

One way the profession holds on to its power is by exercising the privilege of exclusivity granted its members by the state through licensure. Physicians regard exclusivity as a "right."[5] In the United States, courts have ruled that the license is a property right of the physician, not a privilege granted by the people through their elected representatives. Licensure depends not on evidence of beneficial medical practices but on the alleged need to protect the system from pretenders. By licensure, physicians have the right to do as they please and to develop their property as they see fit, including selecting and training new physicians. They have always perceived legislative attempts to alter the economic conditions of medical practice or constrain or change medical practices in other ways as a violation of their fundamental rights.

The courts grant physicians the exclusive right to say who a real doctor is and to establish standards of medical practice without interference from the public. The rationale is that physicians have expertise and special knowledge no one else has and hence are the only people qualified to judge medical matters. (In similar fashion the legal system recognizes no au-

4. R.J. Blendon, "Can China's Health Care Be Transplanted Without China's Economic Policies?" *New England Journal of Medicine* 300(1979):1453.
5. A.R. Jonsen, *The Rights of Physicians*, p. 8.

thority but that of chiropractors to identify a real chiropractor and define acceptable chiropractic practices.) The near absolute belief of the laity in the exclusive right of the profession to judge and regulate itself has made the profession virtually autonomous.

The only real threat to the autonomy of physicians has come from within the ranks, and these doctors criticize the profession at their own risk. Authority based on charismatic or supernatural power always has been susceptible to dissent from within. As a monk preaching fallibility of the doctrine is unwelcome, so is a physician questioning medical practice. Although physicians will in general accept a modicum of internal discussion and controversy as being "healthy," they will brook no physician's criticism that may undermine the faith of the public. Thus, George Crile, Jr., a Cleveland surgeon, was rebuked by the Ethics Committee of the Cleveland Academy of Medicine for expressing in a newspaper interview his opinion that radical mastectomy was archaic and no longer necessary.

The committee did not address the question of the benefit of radical mastectomy, but expressed its concern for "the deleterious effect on the relationship patients have with their surgeons—all different specialties of surgeons—in permitting another obstacle to be erected between the confidence and understanding so necessary for success in an operative procedure."[6] The important point here is that the sanctity of the physician's authority is put above truth and accuracy in medical practice; the well-being of tens of thousands of women who face operations for cancer of the breast is secondary to trust in the doctor.

The closing of the ranks is essential for maintaining the monolithic appearance of authority, and probably explains as well as anything the reluctance of physicians to testify against each other in court. Physicians commonly invoke the sentiment,

6. George Crile, "The Surgeon's Dilemma," *Harper's Magazine* 250(1975):33.

"There but for the grace of God go I," meaning that any physician is bound to make a human mistake sooner or later, and when he does he should not be in jeopardy at the caprice of the courts. There is probably something to this, but it does not uncover a more telling source of reticence. The physician who testifies against another physician is a renegade because he undermines the authority of a colleague, and in so doing exposes the fragile basis of individual authority on which most physicians ultimately depend.

Similarly, the profession will go to any length to avoid public censure of one of its members, no matter the harm being wreaked on innocent patients. Disciplining of physicians by professional societies is done not according to the best interests of the public, but from the perspective of what is best for the profession. It is conservatively estimated that one physician in a hundred needs some sort of discipline every year. Consider the consequences of doing this. Frequent disciplinary decisions would call the public's attention to the fallibility of physicians; the public would discern a higher authority than the individual physician; and the logical next step would be public involvement in setting standards for physicians and enforcing them. Such a policy would be ruinous to the medical profession as it now operates. Far better for the profession to act only if a practitioner's behavior is so detrimental to the professional image that the authority of other practitioners is in greater jeopardy from inaction than from expulsion.

PRICE DETERMINATION IN MEDICINE

In the private sector of medicine, financial transactions are based on an anomaly of free enterprise. There is no competition in the usual sense. If we consider the physician-entrepreneur as a company for descriptive purposes, we find the following characteristics of the business: (1) management and labor are the same; (2) prices are set by the company without the restraints of marketplace competition; (3) the company decides who shall buy and how much; (4) the purchaser doesn't have to pay out of his own pocket (insurance covers most fees), thus assuring the company that almost all of its charges will be paid; (5) the company alone assesses the success of its services and products — the public is deemed ignorant and incapable of judging what it receives; (6) the business is run to maximize the gains of the company, and there is no effective consumerism, public scrutiny or regulation of the business.

There is no other business in our society able to operate under such favorable conditions. The entrepreneurial physician is generously assisted if not genuinely enticed by public largess: The major arena of work (the hospital) is supplied without rent; expensive equipment and instruments are acquired for physicians by hospital administrators who must maintain the image of a modern hospital and staff it with satisfied doctors; research leading to new technologies and treatments is funded from the public till; recruitment and training of new physicians is largely state-supported; supporting personnel (e.g., nurses, technicians, operating room assistants) are paid by the hospital, not the doctor. Society heavily subsidizes its most lucrative profession.

In addition, medical practitioners are able to set prices as high as they wish, within the bounds of what is considered decent within the community. The ordinary rules of the marketplace do not work to keep prices in line with supply and demand. Indeed, it is a common observation that when an area becomes over-populated with physicians, prices actually go up rather than down, because physicians reason that to maintain their incomes they must charge more to compensate for declining business. Because there is no effective price competition, they are able to do this. Furthermore, the number of procedures — e.g., elective operations — is proportional to the number of physicians who can perform them.[7] In contrast to former times, private practice

7. J. Wennberg and A. Gittlesohn, "Small Area Variations in Health Care Delivery," *Science* 182(1973):1102; J.P. Bunker, "Surgical Manpower: A Comparison of Operations and Surgeons in the United States and in England and

fees are now supported by insurance plans, both governmental and private. Just how professional fees are set by insurance providers is a complex affair, but the influence of physicians, both direct and indirect, in setting fees through support of the major insurance carriers in the United States, such as Blue Cross and Blue Shield, is well known.[8] Furthermore, the courts have not held unlawful physicians' pricing schemes that almost surely would have been disallowed under the antitrust laws had the defendants been commercial organizations.

Because such a high proportion of medical expenses is paid by third parties, the individual patient has little incentive to reduce costs. Patients become claimants, not consumers. The result is maximal interest in performing any service or procedure that the individual or his physician thinks may be desirable, whether it is beneficial or not, without regard for the overall interests of society, which foots the bill in the hope of obtaining the best and most efficient medical care for all its citizens.

The fee-for-service system encourages overutilization of services and procedures. Conversely, under prepaid plans or systems where the physician is paid by salary, there may be a tendency to "underutilization" or "underdoctoring," for economic reasons, although to date there is no evidence of this and there are safeguards to prevent it from happening. At the most, a patient might suffer from the insensitivity and indolence of a salaried physician, but never from a conflict of interest, as in the fee-for-service system. One can not say for sure that one financial arrangement is inherently better or worse than another, but only that financial incentives are an important component of medical decision-making.

Economists note the primary role of the physician in control-

Wales," *New England Journal of Medicine* 282(1970):135; E. Vayda, "A Comparison of Surgical Rates in Canada and in England and Wales," *New England Journal of Medicine* 289(1973):1224.

8. J.E. Moss, "Congressional Scrutiny Reveals Sore Spots of U.S. Health Care," *Legal Aspects of Medical Practice* 6(1978):28; Spencer Klaw, *The Great American Medicine Show*, p. 156.

ling medical expenditures of all types, not just professional fees.[9] As Victor Fuchs has put it, the physician is "the captain of the team," who controls almost all medical costs through his decisions about what services to use.[10] While the proportion of medical expenses accounted for by physicians' fees has been stable at about twenty percent,[11] the remaining eighty percent are controlled and often initiated by physicians' decisions. For example, if a physician decides that a patient must enter the hospital for an operation, and the total expense is fifteen thousand dollars, the decision has produced not only approximately three thousand dollars in physician's fees, but the twelve thousand dollars of other expenses accrued in the hospital. With the present practice of doing everything possible for every patient, and usually by the most expensive means, total expenditures are limited only by the amount of money available through government and private insurance sources.

Physicians not only are the key to day-to-day expenses, but they are the major influence in purchases of capital equipment, hospital construction, and the overall financial policies of hospitals. So long as physicians want more hospital beds, or more equipment for each bed, they will find a way of getting it. Probably more than seventy percent of all expenditures for personal health care are the result of decisions of doctors on an individual basis.[12]

The most important fact of medical economics is that we are faced with limited resources for medical expenditures. In North America during the 1960s it seemed as though there were no limits to medical spending, and spending increased at a rapid pace. In the United States from 1950 to 1977, national health expenditures increased from 4.6 to 8.8 percent of the gross

9. A.C. Enthoven, "Cutting Cost Without Cutting the Quality of Care," *New England Journal of Medicine* 298(1978):1229.

10. Victor R. Fuchs, *Who Shall Live?*, p. 57.

11. Enthoven, "Cutting Cost," p. 1229.

12. A.S. Relman, "The Allocation of Medical Resources by Physicians," *Journal of Medical Education* 55(1980):99.

national product, and the figure is now almost 10 percent. Although conceivably the proportion of total resources allocated to medical services could increase even further, expenditures have reached such a high level that there are increasing pressures to stabilize or even reduce medical spending. In virtually all societies there are limited resources for medical spending, and there is a growing consensus in the industrialized countries that further increases in medical expenditures do not bring commensurate benefits, but rather that we have reached a point of medical diminishing returns.[13] Following a period of rapid and dramatic technical advances, we are now in a period in which great expense is required to produce small and questionable technologic gains.

Money still abounds, however, for high-cost technical procedures and intensive-care equipment, the benefits of which are often limited and uncertain. The result is what has been called "halfway technology," the sort of therapy that does not cure but may have some benefit in prolonging life or relieving disability.[14] This sort of technology is extremely expensive, is of dubious efficiency, and does nothing to solve the underlying problem or to prevent the disease. Coronary bypass surgery is an example of a halfway technology vigorously promoted by the medical profession. The $2 billion spent annually on this technology is more than half the entire budget of the National Institutes of Health. Yet, if the money spent on bypass surgery during the last ten years had been spent instead on research aimed at the problem of coronary artery disease, we would by now very possibly know how to prevent this widespread affliction.

By allowing medical resource allocations to be directed by physicians, society allows some services to be excluded in favor of others as surely as this occurs under national health services. There is, in effect, a rationing of services not by a central admin-

13. J.P. Bunker, "When the Medical Interests of Society Are in Conflict with Those of the Individual, Who Wins?" *Pharos* 39(1976):64.
14. Lewis Thomas, *Lives of a Cell*, p. 37.

istration, but by the choices of physicians. Thus, in America, high-technology medicine is available to most people, but child and maternal care and home services are lacking for large segments of the population. Hospitals often have insufficient funds for adequate nurse staffing, the status of nursing homes is a national disgrace, and rehabilitation and preventive medicine programs are underfunded.

Those who look seriously at health care on a societal level conclude that the real gains in health, both historically and now, are from preventive medicine applied on a communitywide scale—e.g., nutrition, sanitation and a healthful environment.[15] (See Chapter 7.) Thus, the greater benefits to society do not come from individual treatment by doctors. Most truly curative therapies, such as penicillin and polio vaccine, have come from research. As expenditures for prevention, including research, are five percent or less of all medical expenditures,[16] the funneling of resources into individual-treatment medicine is contrary to the greater societal interest.

One must remember that no matter how the medical pie is sliced, allocations to medicine come from the larger resources of society. During the period when medical expenditures have more than doubled as a proportion of the U.S. gross national product, increased payroll deductions and personal expenditures for medical services have left less to spend for other goods and services, and increased governmental medical spending within a limited budget has meant less for other programs. The medical profession is able to increase resources allocated to it by combining research on high-cost technology with the demand that all citizens by given full access to this sort of " big medicine," along with the stipulation that someone else pay for it. With a burgeoning technology such as radioisotope scanning, the profession can divert millions of dollars of additional spend-

15. Steven Jonas, *Medical Mystery*, pp. 49, 51; Thomas McKeown, *The Role of Medicine*, pp. 71-113.
16. Jonas, *Medical Mystery*, p. 60.

ing to the medical sector by the simple expedient of saying that patients must have the service, even without evidence of benefit.[17]

Acquisition of the new technologies is a social and professional necessity for physicians and hospitals, none of which want to appear "behind" in medical practice. The cost of reproducing scanners and ultrasound machines in every hospital is prodigious, and as the cost is passed on to the consumer, the insurance companies and welfare agencies end up paying for faddish gadgets and the playthings of physicians. While the medical profession is given the power to assert what should be spent on its services and takes full advantage of insurance systems that reward those who spend the most, those who want money for prison reform or for virtually any other public service, must compete for public funding by demonstrating need and benefit to the community.

As a result, medicine is now receiving a larger share of society's resources. Whether this is advantageous for the public is a moot question; what is clear is that the public has had nothing to say about it. In countries in which medical spending is controlled through allocations to national health insurance, there is public participation in deciding how much will go to medicine instead of to other social services, to support of industries or even to military defense. Under the present private medical system there is no public choice because the medical profession alone decides the extent of expenditures. Certainly the members of any profession are the ones in the best position to provide the information necessary to make informed and equitable choices; that is not at question. The question is whether those professionals alone should be allowed to make economic decisions that are inevitably biased toward serving the interests of the profession, without consulting those who are paying the bill.

It is in the public interest to understand the far-reaching as-

17. G.E. Burch, "Of 'Now Myocardial Imaging,'" *American Heart Journal* 99(1980):540.

pects of the system of medical economics and how any economic system affects any individual's medical care. As individuals, we all tend to believe that the sort of medical care we receive is what is uniquely best for us, irrespective of financial considerations. Or we believe that if we are resourceful enough to choose a good doctor whose integrity can be trusted to protect us, economic factors will not be an issue. Unfortunately, this is not and can not be the case. The honest physician can try to minimize costs, but the location of his office, the equipment he uses, and the very standards of practice he takes as a starting point are determined in an important way by the financial system within which he works.

If we no longer accept the ancient view that health is the privilege of the rich, and believe that the practice of medicine should follow the ideal of giving as much caring and curing to as many persons as possible by use of our skills and scientific knowledge, we must eliminate those factors that detract from the ideal. It seems tragic that a profession that makes claim to the lofty ideals of service to mankind should fall short of its potential because of the distortions of economic interests that in turn distort medical practices, distribution of resources, and the covenant between doctor and patient.

DEFINING SOCIAL ISSUES AS MEDICAL PROBLEMS

> As long as the public bows to the professional monopoly in assigning the sick-role, it cannot control hidden health hierarchies that multiply patients. The medical clergy can be controlled only if the law is used to restrict and disestablish its monopoly on deciding what constitutes disease, who is sick, and what ought to be done to him or her.
>
> Ivan Illich,
> *Medical Nemesis*

The unwritten contract between society and the medical profession gives physicians the authority to define health, to label one person's illness legitimate disease, to deny that another person's illness is a real disease, and to pronounce diseased a third person who has no complaint of illness. Many writers speak of "the medicalization of social problems," by which they mean the power of the medical profession to define a medical problem and decide how society should view the problem, as well as how it should be treated.[18]

The attitude that makes this possible is evident in our language when we use phrases such as "He's sick," or "This policy is a cancer within the department" to describe people or things we don't like. Disease becomes a metaphor for socially undesirable conditions, and by failing to distinguish between biological dysfunction and social taboo, society gives the medical profession as much power over social and moral decisions as it gives to judges and schoolteachers. In allowing medical jurisdiction over matters such as drug addiction, or when and where a person should be allowed to die, the public relinquishes control over decisions that physicians are no more qualified to make than anyone else. Perhaps the preference for medical solutions is the easy way out of tough social problems, but the public should be aware that in disowning social responsibilities it increases the power of the medical profession to create illness by defining it—a form of iatrogenesis—and to treat it according to the interests and needs of the profession, which may be distinctly different from the interests and needs of the "patients" and the public.

If homosexuality, for instance, is defined as a disease, the resolution of what are essentially social concerns falls under the jurisdiction of the medical profession, and solutions are more likely to reflect professional interests and standards than those of the larger society or the individuals involved. Similarly, for the essentially social problem of care of the elderly, society chooses the medical solution of nursing homes. The care and treatment of the elderly are therefore controlled by medical

18. Eliot Freidson, *Profession of Medicine*, p. 20; David Mechanic, *Future Issues in Health Care*, p. 146; Ivan Illich, *Medical Nemesis*, p. 37.

professionals and not by family and friends. Although many physicians do not welcome this expanded jurisdiction, they are called upon to determine what will be done about alcoholism or rape or alleged mental illness in persons who have committed criminal acts. The public has lost, if indeed it ever had, the right to evaluate its own behavior, the right to decide what illness should be left alone or tended to by families, and the right to decide who should be in hospitals and who should not. Indeed, it has lost the very right to negotiate the conditions under which it submits to the authority of medical professionals.

THE POLITICAL NATURE OF MEDICINE

> Medicine is a social science and politics are nothing else than medicine on a large scale.
>
>   Rudolf Virchow

Unlike the school system, the court system, penal institutions, and even such esoteric and technical fields as space exploration and national defense, medicine is seldom examined from a political perspective, or from the perspective of informed consumers. It is one of the parodoxes of modern society that a public service accounting for about ten percent of the nation's economic expenditures, holding control over the health and well-being of almost every citizen, and affecting society at every level, should have almost no public participation in or control of its workings. By any rational analysis, when individuals and society have a large stake in anything, their opinion and needs should determine policies and practices.

The Director-General of the World Health Organization has pointed out the need for public involvement in medicine:

> What I am advocating, for the industrial as well as the developing world, is for the health establishment to make a major effort to describe all the health problems and the alternative ways of dealing with them in an objective way and then to accept a national decision process based upon this evidence. Such a series of steps has risks as well as advantages and assumes both a level of

scientific detachment which is clearly obvious to all and an acceptance that the final decisions are made by society rather than by the concerned professionals.[19]

Even within the medical profession there are some who believe that society should make the final decisions on medical policy, as is obvious from the following statement extracted from a report of the Committee on Ethics of the American Heart Association:

> A scientist's work and, indeed, his/her very qualifications are products of an extensive and overlapping series of franchises conferred by society . . . . Society is only now beginning to recognize the extent of such franchises and to be aware of levels of accountability beyond what has been customary. Society can legitimately expect a role in stating need and in setting priorities for research and application at all levels . . . . Not only is there responsibility to fulfill the public's right to know, but also responsibility to contribute to the pluralistic decision in social policy that the public may want to make . . . . The judgment of what is of value to the public is a proper concern of that public and cannot be left exclusively to the scientific subcommunity.[20]

Certainly, issues such as national health insurance and health planning of any sort require public participation, without which the profession would be given unimaginable license supported by public funding. Many of the public view the issue of national health insurance as a strictly economic one, in which the only problem is how to obtain access to medical care for all persons without imposing financial hardship on anyone. This is certainly an important matter, but it is narrow, for it focuses only on how we will finance our medical system and not on what our medical system will be. But even in the narrower sense, any effort to contain or restrain medical spending requires more than medical expertise; it requires a political dialogue involving the

19. H. Mahler, "Health—A Demystification of Medical Technology," *Lancet* 2(1975):829.

20. "An Ethical Consideration of Large-Scale Clinical Trials in Cardiovascular Diseases," *Circulation* 52(1975):page 5.

public. Whether the political process results in a barefoot doctor in China, a salaried physician in England, or a fee-for-service practitioner in North America, the important point is that the type of practice is a reflection of the political environment in which it is carried out. In a democratic society, there is a responsibility, if not actually a requirement, that private citizens and groups representing those citizens become involved in decisions whose consequences affect them. In the Western democracies it is incongruous for the public to be excluded from setting medical policy.

PUBLIC INVOLVEMENT IN MEDICINE

While physicians and others who provide medical services are well organized and able to manipulate government and individuals in the interests of their guilds and themselves, in effect plundering the public treasury, consumers are poorly organized and relatively ineffective in trying to counter the power of medical providers.

As they perceive that their interests are at stake with regard to nuclear power and industrial uses of toxic chemicals and waste products, private individuals and public interest groups have become a potent political force in directing policy in these fields, and even in instances where the public concern is of a medical nature, such as exposure to low-level radiation, the public will react so long as the medical profession is not directly involved. For example, a controversial study showed that an abnormally high number of workers employed at a complex of nuclear power plants in the western United States had died of cancer of the pancreas, lung and bone.[21] The findings so infuriated several labor unions that they demanded that the Secretary of the Department of Health, Education and Welfare do something about it. In the celebrated case of Karen Silkwood, a worker in a

21. "Hanford and the Radiation Report," The Weekly (Seattle), March 7, 1979, p. 4.

nuclear power plant in Oklahoma who died in an automobile accident a week after being contaminated with plutonium, the entire nuclear power industry was made accountable through the courts for the medical safety of all exposed persons. Safeguards for employees against occupational health hazards are openly negotiated in virtually every industry.

But unlike the healthy and democratic inquiry that gets action in cases where industrial and governmental policies and practices are seen to affect the health of the citizenry, there is an almost total absence of such inquiry into the effects of medical policies and practices on the health of the people, even though the magnitude of health problems created by industry and government shrinks when viewed beside those originating within the medical profession.

If nuclear radiation leaks cause cancer, the number who die from it is a small fraction of the number of women who get vaginal cancer because their mothers were given diethylstilbestrol by their physicians during pregnancy.[22] Why is there not a proportionately greater public outcry over the tragedy of that medical abuse? Why is there no public inquiry into the circumstances, practices and professional attitudes that not only allow such a tragedy, but actually spawn it? During the early years of heart transplantation and coronary bypass surgery, when those procedures were experimental in every sense, and the mortality from the procedures exceeded that of leaving patients alone, why were there no labor unions or consumer groups up in arms over the suffering and death that resulted? Why, in a democracy with a free press, was the public largely unaware of these problems and indifferent to the few reports of them?

When consumers will fight a five-percent rate hike in the cost of natural gas, or boycott beef because of high prices, how do we explain public apathy over increases of twenty-nine to seventy-five percent in surgeons' fees for common procedures over a

22. M. Bibbo, "Follow-Up Study of Male and Female Offspring of DES-Exposed Mothers," *Journal of Obstetrics and Gynecology* 49(1977):1.

three-year period?[23] When governmental policies concerning schools, police departments and public parks are scrutinized in order to protect the common interest, why is the citizenry so ill-informed that harmful medical practices and treatments can come and go in faddist cycles that would make any clothier drool? The public is content to wear the medical fashion of the day without asking the price or the quality of the material, and indeed often not even knowing what it is wearing. Is there any other industry in which the purported good intentions of the seller are sufficient to still the demands of the buyer for just return?

There are, in fact, some consumer groups working in the medical field, and although they deserve credit for attempting to do what few have any appetite for, they are severely limited by insufficient funds and the indifference of the people they represent. Furthermore, they restrict themselves to pecking at the outside of the system rather than going to the core of the problem. Attempts to reform medical care are directed not at decisive practices but at the embroidery. Similarly, governmental agencies are now attempting to assess the results of medical technology, a new step in medical consumerism that is anathema to the medical profession. To make such assessments the agencies must rely on information supplied by physicians. For instance, to find out whether hysterectomy improves health, the researcher needs data from physicians about the benefits and ill-effects of the procedure; but this information does not exist because physicians have not obtained it in a systematic manner.[24] An assessment of coronary bypass surgery is totally dependent on the manner in which physicians measure and report the results of that operation, and unless independent agencies

23. T.L. Delbanco, K.C. Meyers and E.A. Segal, "Paying the Physician's Fee," *New England Journal of Medicine* 301(1979):1314.

24. U.S. Office of Technology Assessment, *Assessing the Efficacy and Safety of Medical Technologies* (Washington, D.C.: Government Printing Office, 1978), p. 47.

do the actual measuring, no one can effectively challenge the conclusions of the medical profession.

The trouble with most medical consumer groups is that they do not question the source of medical decisions and policy, the physicians, and they restrict their concerns to better and more humane care of patients through present professional practices — pressing for improved staffing, better waiting rooms, better access to medical facilities and more comprehensive services, elimination of worthless or harmful drugs, and patients' rights programs. These are all worthy pursuits, but just as covering a bad steak with sauce may make it more palatable, these efforts do not get at the source of the problem, the physician himself. Medical reform can come only through changing those who practice medicine, because reform must be in the practice itself, not in how it is distributed.

Why is there so little consumer participation in medicine? First and foremost, consumerism is antithetical to the basic contract and the therapeutic relationship. Consumerism is not compatible with the idea of a healer possessed of special powers. Second, the public is apathetic. Despite the erosion of confidence in doctors, people generally are satisfied with medical care, even if they have complaints about one aspect or another. But apathy is not explanation enough; there is apathy about food prices and the cost of gasoline until the public perceives that its interests are being trampled. In the area of medicine, public indifference arises from ignorance of medical issues. Consumer ignorance is a source of monopoly power in any field, and in the industrialized countries the consumer is nowhere as ignorant as in purchases of medical services. As we have seen, the consumer is seldom the person who makes the decision to purchase, he knows little of what is being ordered for him, and he is relatively powerless to confront the physician over decisions. In addition, it is not at all clear that patients want to make the important decisions and confrontations necessary to become effective medical consumerists. They do not believe they are qualified to judge medical affairs.

Notice, for instance, the statement of Felix Frankfurter quoted at the beginning of this chapter. If a justice of the U.S. Supreme Court proclaims that, "I am not competent to have any views on the very difficult problem of the relations between the medical profession and society,"[25] who, we may ask, is? The public, including lawyers, must realize that they are not only qualified to make decisions involving nonbiological matters arising in medical affairs, but that they injure themselves by not doing so.

The law and its courts have avoided attempts to introduce public policy into medical practices. In negligence cases the courts have upheld, with rare exceptions, the doctrine that standard of care is defined by the profession, not the public, that the establishment of medical practice is the domain of physicians alone. The courts do not judge the benefit or harm of a practice, but only whether it conforms to the standards of the professional group doing it. Thus malpractice means only that the physician has failed to exercise the degree of skill and learning commonly applied by the average prudent and reputable member of the profession. If a patient suffers harm from an untested and unproven treatment, the courts find no negligence if it is standard or acceptable to the medical profession. The physician is at risk only when he deviates from his guild's rules. A plaintiff's lawyer has no chance of winning judgment against a physician unless another physician is willing to testify that the act under question was not "good medical practice."

Even by this restricted definition of malpractice, most patients who are victims of it are not compensated for their loss, being unaware that they are victims, as most iatrogenic harm is hidden under the claim of unavoidable side effects of necessary treatment. As often as not, the patient expresses profound gratitude to the offending doctor who is perceived as having done the best possible job under the circumstances. No one is witness to the

25. Felix Frankfurter, "A Lawyer's Dicta on Doctors," p. 17.

ultimate harm. As Molière's "Reluctant Doctor" Sganarelle said, "We never make mistakes. It's always the corpse's fault. And the best of it is, dead men are very decent sort of folk. You never hear them complain of the doctors who killed them."

But more far-reaching than the ineffectuality of lawsuits to compensate most of the people who have suffered from malpractice is the total inability of the legal process to allow public participation in medicine. Malpractice suits do not question the authority or autonomy of the physician; they do not challenge the infallibility of physicians' judgments in areas of professional uncertainty; they do not question the public benefit of standard medical practices; they do not introduce public involvement in setting standards of medical practices. By the medium of malpractice suits the public ironically enforces the autonomy and exclusivity of the medical profession in determining medical practices.

The courts accord special privileges to physicians in absolving them from the responsibility of acting in the public interest because lawmakers have placed the domain of medicine outside the public jurisdiction, in keeping with the basic contract. The collusion between profession and public in maintaining the autonomy of the physician precludes any effective consumerism, and until there is a conceptual change in the minds of the public or the profession or both, there can be no challenge to basic medical practices strong enough to bring about reform.

The ability of consumer or governmental action to alter the practice of medicine is beyond dispute. Although perhaps not perceived as such, the control of medical abortions through public policy is an example of extremely effective consumerism. The abortion issue is an extraordinary instance of popular insistence that a particular medical procedure should not fall under the exclusive jurisdiction of medical professionals. The public has taken exclusive control of abortion away from doctors, through various statutes dictating when it may be performed and whether the public will pay for it. The abortion issue is treated this way because the public perceives it not as a medical matter but as a social or religious concern. This demonstrates that when the public perceives a medical practice as impinging on basic human values expressed in social and religious terms, it is not only willing to act, but assumes its usual aggressive posture in demanding this or that action. Interestingly, the public does not see the abortion issue vis-à-vis the medical profession, but rather as a fight among special-interest groups.

Even the U.S. Supreme Court, in limiting Medicaid payments for abortions to cases in which the life of the mother is endangered, or to cases of promptly reported rape or incest, made a distinction between abortions and other medical procedures. "Abortion is inherently different from other medical procedures," in the opinion of the court, "because no other procedure involves the purposeful termination of a potential life."[26] By this pronouncement the Supreme Court allowed itself jurisdiction over a medical procedure by labeling it nonmedical. But the deeper meaning of the abortion issue is that once the public perceives that its interests are involved, it has the power to alter medical practices.

If abortion is a legitimate social concern subject to public control, why is dying in hospitals or the use of unproven therapies not an equally legitimate concern? Consumers need to address the basic questions of medical policy and practice, which means questioning the assumptions and special status of physicians. Consumers must consider their priorities for spending money on procedures and spending it on more basic medical needs such as nutrition and prevention of chronic diseases; they must realize that high medical expenditures mean less public money for other social and economic needs; they must question whether any medical practice is of benefit to those who receive it. Organizations as well as individuals must challenge the medical monopoly. Corporations and unions, which pay two thousand dollars or more a year per worker for health insurance,

26. Harris v. McRae, 40 C.C.H. Supreme Court Bull., pp. B4021-82.

should be vitally interested in altering medical programs and practices so as to decrease the subsidy to the medical enterprise. General Motors pays more each year to Michigan Blue Cross/ Blue Shield than it does to U.S. Steel.

Although the consumer must have the power to negotiate with the supplier, the danger of substituting the will of the consumer for professional expertise must be acknowledged. There is already enough individual consumerism in the form of pressure on physicians and hospitals to use new technologies as soon as they are publicly known, as well as popular but nonbeneficial medical practices, to give rise to concern that rampant consumerism could reduce medical practice to fulfilling the whims of an uninformed public. If physicians had to practice according to the desires, not the needs, of the public, they would soon be operating like the itinerant quack who supplies the cure for every need. The self-interests of consumer groups can be as destructive and tyrannical as those of any autonomous profession. If we want the physician to be more than a mere servant of the public conception of what is needed, we must use his expertise wisely; otherwise there is little point in obtaining a professional service. What we are striving for is a healthy balance between suppliers and consumers, seeking neither professional elitism nor a public disregard for professional expertise.

APPROACHES TO CHANGE

In the present circumstances of professional dominance over policy, there are three approaches to change in medicine: The first two, internal regulation by the profession and external regulation by the government are, in varying mixes, tried in almost all countries. The third, the one that could work, is a prerequisite change in the attitudes of physicians and healers on the one hand, and the consuming public on the other, which would alter the basic physician-patient contract so as to reorient medical practices to the needs of individual patients and the body politic.

A key element in the basic contract is the physician's obligation to regulate his professional behavior himself so that it will
coincide with the needs and desires of his patients. Perhaps
there was a time when, as individual dealing with individual,
the physician was fully constrained by need for the good will of
the patient. But with the complexity of modern medical
technology and the distortions of medical financing, self-
regulation has become a matter of self-discipline and protection
of the professional guild. There is no patient-oriented professional self-regulation. Physicians individually and collectively
do not regulate medical costs or physicians' fees (the prime
determinant of medical costs); they do not regulate treatments
and procedures for safety and benefit; they resist efforts to set
standards and monitor quality (peer review has been ineffective
by all accounts); and above all, they resist any attempt even from
within the profession to regulate the actual practices of individual physicians. Through specialty certification the profession regulates who may perform certain practices, but there is no
regulation of the practices themselves.

A grim consequence of the failure of internal regulation occurred in 1969 when Dr. Denton Cooley implanted the first
artificial heart into a human being, although experiments with
the heart on animals had been disastrous, and the developers of
the heart (who did not know of Dr. Cooley's intended use of it)
considered it not fit for human use.[27] By all scientific standards,
use of the artificial heart was experimental, and the patient who
unwittingly received it died shortly thereafter. In responding to
criticisms that he had not submitted a protocol for the experiment to the Baylor College of Medicine Faculty Committee on
Research Involving Human Beings, nor had he abided by the
guidelines of the National Heart Institute which had supplied

27. Renee C. Fox and Judith P. Swazey, *The Courage to Fail*, pp. 149-211. The
incident evoked a bitter dispute between Dr. Michael DeBakey, developer of the
heart, and Dr. Cooley. Without notifying DeBakey, Cooley hired DeBakey's en-
gineer, who supplied Cooley with one of the hearts.

funds for development of the artificial heart, Cooley said:

> I have done more heart surgery than anyone else in the world.
> Based on this experience, I believe I am qualified to judge what is
> right and proper for my patients. The permission I receive to do
> what I do I receive from my patients. It is not received from a
> government agency or one of my seniors.[28]

Although a less celebrated medical personality might not
have escaped unscathed from such a misadventure, it nevertheless represents the extreme expression of physician autonomy
and disdain for any regulation the individual physician deems
inappropriate, and the profession acquiesces in this attitude,
which marks not only the spirit of "medical freedom" by which
physicians assume the right to do whatever they see fit, but the
ultimate rejection in one clean sweep of both internal and external regulation. Thus, the physician's idea of regulation does not
derive from the notion of submission to a higher authority acting
in the interests of, or even in negotiation with, the other party,
but ultimately resides in the concept that what the physician
does is best for the patient.

This concept is enshrouded in the pervading professional
belief that the profession does regulate itself in time, which is a
restatement of the belief in and desire for professional autonomy.
But by the very nature of the profession, and its intent to serve
itself and maintain the privileged position of its members, it can
not regulate itself because it believes in its own vitality and
correctness and does not represent the public with which it is in
contractual agreement. As George Bernard Shaw said, "All professions are conspiracies against the laity."[29] We are better off
recognizing and dealing with this fact than naively hoping for
internal professional regulation.

Although external regulation, mostly by governmental agencies, has been successful in representing the public need in some

28. Fox and Swazey, *The Courage to Fail*, p. 190.
29. George Bernard Shaw, *The Doctor's Dilemma*, p. 116.

areas, particularly drugs, this form of regulation has distinct limitations. It is expensive, monitoring the behavior of physicians with respect to standards is impossible (especially when there are no standards), government regulation is subject to political influences, it is essentially a negative incentive and therefore requires policing, and its consequences are always somewhat different from what is expected.

The courts, while shrinking from curbing the power of the profession to dictate medical practices, have exercised a kind of external regulation by recognizing and repeatedly affirming the responsibility of the state to help individuals who can not protect themselves in medical matters. In the second case to reach the U.S. Supreme Court under the Federal Food, Drug, and Cosmetic Act of 1938, Justice Frankfurter said:

> Congress extended the range of its control over illicit and noxious articles and stiffened the penalties for disobedience. The purposes of this legislation thus touch phases of the lives and health of people which, in the circumstances of modern industrialism, are largely beyond self-protection.[30]

Although the legislation applied only to drugs, and very recently to medical devices, the court affirmed the intent of the law to protect individuals from "the circumstances of modern industrialization," to wit the technological and social structure of medicine before which the individual is relatively helpless. In a prior case, the judge stated that the purpose of the 1938 act was "to protect the public, the vast multitude which includes the ignorant, the unthinking, and the credulous who, when making a purchase, do not stop to analyze."[31] This includes all of us.

Legislators and jurists, in obeisance to the basic doctor-patient contract, however, are unwilling to apply the principle of protection to medical professional practices. While drugs are strictly regulated with respect to standards and content, there is no restriction on uses by a physician once the drug is approved.

30. U.S. v Dotterweich, 320 U.S. 227, in *Kleinfeld and Dunn* (1938-49), p. 280.
31. Cited in James H. Young, *The Medical Messiahs*, pp. 210-15.

Thus, an antibiotic may be deemed safe and beneficial for certain uses, but there is no way to force doctors to use it appropriately. Objects, such as drugs, pacemakers and even hospital buildings, can be regulated, but how a doctor uses a drug or hospital is a practice. Similarly, operations and other procedures are practices, and so have always been exempted from external regulation. Not only is there no law to ensure the proper use of an operation, but there is not even a requirement that the operation be proved safe and beneficial under optimal conditions. There is, in short, no FDA for surgeons.

It is irrational to regulate drugs in the public interest and not to apply the same logic to surgical procedures that are, by their very nature, potentially more harmful and therefore more in need of regulation. This disparity reflects the public's belief in the sanctity of the physician's practices.

Despite the protection afforded the medical profession by the law, there is clear evidence of the beginnings of change. Recent court decisions show that the legal system does have an interest in altering the doctor-patient relationship in favor of the patient. The expanding idea of informed consent makes it clear that the courts and the legislatures in some instances are concerned with the rights of patients to have access to information, to participate in decisions, and to exercise choices with respect to whether procedures should be performed. Courts have intervened in medical practices in decisions involving sterilization, birth control, and the rights of patients to control their own bodies. In rare cases courts have ruled that in certain circumstances the standard of medical care must be defined by courts rather than by the medical profession. Although the process is slow and is being countered by extreme resistance from the medical profession, the law is a powerful means of redirecting medical practices in accordance with social policies and the public perspective. Public interest groups and, above all, lawyers themselves, must perceive that medical policy is social policy, and that the legal system must act in the public interest.

Public groups such as corporations, unions, governments, and the members of health maintenance organizations and insurance groups such as Blue Cross should insist on some voice in how their dollars are spent and how medical policies are set. These groups should insist upon unbiased evaluations of new medical technologies before they are widely disseminated, and in particular they should call a halt to the practice of third-party payment for unproven therapies or practices. They should ask for environmental impact studies of new medical technologies, so that the public might rightly decide whether alleged benefits outweigh economic, social and bodily costs. They should ask that medical expenditures reflect the proportion of benefit the public receives from preventive medicine and medical research compared to the benefit of encounter medicine.

I do not want to be misinterpreted on this point. High quality curative services are absolutely essential, but high-cost technologically oriented palliative medicine only results in still higher costs, little benefit and too much harm. Public groups should ask for scientific validation of all new medical practices so that the laity can differentiate between the advances of medical science and the claims of quacks and healers.

Physicians will change their practices only if they perceive a public insistence to do so. They will not become more accountable to the public until there is a change in public attitude; accountability under the basic contract can not be legislated. But physicians are capable of change. Already, many physicians are working hard within the medical establishment to make medicine more responsive to patients. Although these men and women are in the minority, most physicians would change if given the proper incentives.

But changes in medicine will come very slowly, for the power, prestige and wealth of physicians is too great to allow for easy change. As in other fields of consumerism, pressures for change often are most effectively applied through groups. The public, individually and collectively, must recognize its stake in health care and voice its wishes through contemporary methods of public policy-making. The goal is not to destroy or reject modern medicine, but to celebrate it and strive to reach its full potential. The one true miracle in medicine was the ascension of Hippocrates, who led physicians away from superstition toward scientific inquiry. The Second Coming of Hippocrates will not appear as a miracle, but must come from the full expression of an informed public using its medical resources for the public good and for the good of individual patients.

CHAPTER TEN

Individual Responsibility for Health Care

> Over 99 per cent of us are born healthy and made sick as a result of personal misbehavior and environmental conditions. The solution to ill health in modern (American) society involves individual responsibility, in the first instance, and social responsibility through public legislative and private voluntary efforts, in the second instance.
>
> John Knowles,
> *Doing Better and Feeling Worse*

> The fact that most individuals unhesitatingly entrust their bodies and lives to doctors about whom they know nothing is a remarkable testimony to the power of social conventions and etiquette. For it demonstrates that even our most supposedly spontaneous responses, those involving trust and mistrust, are ultimately felt, not according to "authentic inner" experiences, but rather according to frameworks of social reality and behavioral properties that are created and sustained by organizations and institutions.
>
> Marcia Millman,
> *The Unkindest Cut*

IF IT IS true, as argued earlier, that health is much less a function of patient-physician encounters and medical intervention than it is a matter of nutrition, good personal health habits, sanitation, and environmental elements, it follows that primary responsibility for control of those factors rests not with the medical profession but with individuals and nonmedical organizations. Physicians can and should be expert advisors in coping with individual health problems, but they can not alone provide health. Governments and corporations are perhaps remiss in not providing greater protection from environmental hazards, but public agencies can not be responsible for individual health habits.

Contrary to the popular belief that we become sick and are made well, smoking, overeating, sedentary habits, alcohol and drug abuse, use of handguns (the primary cause of death of young men in the central cities), unsafe driving habits, and inability to control stress are more the villains of poor health and death in modern society than deprivation of adequate medical care. The person who disregards these factors while expecting health to come from other sources is acting inhumanely toward himself. All persons have a right to access to appropriate medical expertise, but the right to health is illusory; no social program can guarantee health.

SELF-CARE

The concept of responsibility for one's own health leads to self-care, the oldest means of health care. The self-care movement ranges from activist patients who work within the conventional medical system to those who reject Western medicine entirely and turn to yoga, meditation, "natural" foods, and an occasional visit to the naturopath. The woman who chooses natural childbirth with medical supervision, the man who takes his own blood pressure at home and the person in a supervised rehabilitation program are all practicing self-care within the context of conventional medicine. Outside of conventional medicine self-care takes many forms, including biofeedback, psychic healing, nutrition, regulation of stress, physical fitness, body therapies, meditation, chiropractic, religion, and all practices designed to provide a healthy personal environment.

The purpose of self-care is to promote health and prevent disease, but in the narrower context this is simply a matter of using common-sense health habits, including not smoking or overeating. The contemporary self-care movement, when viewed as an option to conventional medicine, as it often is, has clear social and political ramifications, and is in part an antagonistic response to conventional medicine and physicians. It is part of the antiestablishment mood of the time, the disillusionment with the cost, toxicity and dehumanization of high-technology medicine, and partially a passive (and aggressive) reaction to the arrogance and power of physicians. Indeed, the popularity of alternative strategies may be in proportion to the increasingly negative public image of the physician as one whose interests and skills are frequently applied with disregard for the emotional needs of the laity.

The movement is to some extent an ideological rejection of modern medicine by persons who may be unaware of the complexities of medical practices and who may be unable to articulate their disagreements, but who seek a return to what they consider to be more basic human values. The "holistic" self-care movement is an expression of the desire for independence and rejection of impersonal technology, the narrowness of the biophysical "fix," and dependence on the physician. As Illich says, under conventional medicine, people "want to be taught, moved, treated, or guided rather than to learn, to heal, and to find their own way."[1] Although there is no evidence that the really important elements of self-care are better attended to by rejecting conventional medicine, the person who wants to learn, to heal, and to find his own way is sometimes better able to do so through an alternative health strategy. Responsible persons will practice self-care whether in a conventional or unconventional setting, but the need to express independence of the domination of biophysical medicine gives meaning to an organized movement.

The self-care movement brings many persons closer to what they consider a more desirable life-philosophy. When self-care is part of an encompassing belief system such as that of psychic healers, it is essential to maintenance of the belief. For many

1. Ivan Illich, *Medical Nemesis,* p. 210.

others, self-care is the means of escaping the domination and impersonality of industrialization and returning to a more "natural" way of life. The reliance on nutrition as the basis of self-care, in addition to promoting the notion of control over one's health, is at the same time a means of rejecting the social policies of the giant food processors and encouraging more simple life habits. "You are what you eat" is a slogan which promotes the comforting notion that one's destiny is literally within one's own hands, but it might be as true to say "You eat what you are." People express, through eating, their philosophies and social beliefs, all of which often have very little to do with the nutritional value of food, much less with specific nutritional needs. Millions of people eat honey instead of refined sugar, because it looks and seems more natural than the processed sugar, but once inside the body they both turn into the same thing.[2] In this example self-care is illusory, and is really little more than a statement of personal social values. If self-care is to be more than a social statement, it must undergo the same rigorous scrutiny we have asked of conventional medicine.

There are, unfortunately, some real and important limitations to self-care. The first important limitation is that on occasion, for most persons, truly curative therapy is necessary, and total reliance on self-care may preclude access to such treatment. Who, for instance, would want to practice self-care on a ruptured appendix? Or diabetic coma, or severe trauma suffered in an

2. Honey, a pleasant natural food, has acquired a reputation for being a medicine and an especially nutritious food. Unfortunately, it is not a medicine and it is no more nutritious than refined table sugar. Honey is about twenty percent water, the remainder consisting mostly of two monosaccharides, glucose and fructose, the only two sugars the body uses in any quantity for energy. Honey contains only traces of other nutrients. Refined table sugar is practically a hundred percent sucrose, which is a disaccharide made of glucose and fructose. Once inside the body, sucrose is broken into glucose and fructose. One tablespoon of honey is converted into sixty-four calories, approximately one-third more than an equal serving of table sugar, and it contains slightly more sodium than sugar does. (Too much sodium causes high blood pressure and heart failure.) Brown sugar is less highly refined sucrose containing traces of other sugars, minerals and coloring substance.

accident, or a bad burn? No rational or sane person would deny the ability of Western medicine to cure certain conditions not curable by other methods, and the immediate problem of self-care is in knowing when to seek expert medical assistance.

Potentially one of the most dangerous concepts is the notion that certain home remedies will cure or prevent all diseases. The claim, for instance, that ascorbic acid (vitamin C) can control virtually all diseases, if taken as fact, would dissuade persons from seeking medical attention when it is necessary. Persons practicing self-care are faced with either disregarding physicians entirely, which is the case with some religious groups (occasionally with fatal consequences), or deciding when someone else's expertise is needed. It may be that eighty to ninety percent of illnesses do not require the attention of a physician, but how is the person practicing self-care to know which do and which do not? The person who attempts to treat presumed diseases might soon be overmedicating himself and creating more bodily and emotional harm than would result from conventional treatment. Furthermore, certain methods of self-care may actually result in more, not fewer, encounters with physicians. In one study of a consumer's guide to self-care, it was demonstrated that if patients with acute viral illnesses had followed the recommendations of the guidebook for when to see a doctor, they would have made more visits to the doctor than they actually did.[3] The value of self-care depends on how one defines it: If by self-care one means avoidance of health risks (e.g., smoking), there is no problem; if by self-care one means treatment of one's own diseases, then there is a serious problem in knowing when to seek professional help, and from whom. To the extent that self-care prevents diseases, it is sensible and beneficial, but beyond that point it is detrimental because it limits its devotees to what can be accomplished without professional expertise.

3. A.O. Berg and J.P. LoGerfo, "Potential Effect of Self-Care on the Number of Physician Visits," *New England Journal of Medicine* 300(1979):535.

Coexisting with the concept of self-care espoused by psychics, many religious groups, and more recently by groups promoting self-fulfillment, is the parallel concept of an individual's responsibility for his own diseases as well as his own health. The notion that patients bring illness on themselves has long been part of Eastern religions and is a part of the holistic concept that health and illness reflect unity or lack of unity in the psyche, the body and the surrounding universe. Just as healing is seen as achieving harmony between mind and body, so disease demonstrates failure to do so. According to this belief, the psyche regulates the body, and the individual controls his or her state of health through control over the psyche. This leads to the belief that diseases are caused by the unconscious willing of the ill person and can be cured by will power or positive thinking, or by integration of the self, or by unity with God.

The idea of disease as an expression of a person's personality or unconscious desires has led to theories of types of persons who are more likely to contract particular diseases. In earlier times tuberculosis was thought to be a disease of dropouts or Bohemians, or of people who had repressed sexual desires and thwarted hopes.[4] Today cancer is believed to be due to despair, loss of a close relationship, low self-esteem, inability to express oneself, and repressed rage.[5] In neither case is there any scientific evidence that the assigned personality traits are more common in persons with the disease than in persons with other diseases. Nor have the promoters of these notions taken into account the real possibility that tuberculosis or cancer precipitates despair or repression of rage in those who contract them.

However, these myths of psychological causes of diseases and responsibility for one's own illness do serve some important social functions related to healing. First, the belief in responsibility for one's own disease allows the patient to assume that he has control over the disease. As discussed before, loss of control

4. Susan Sontag, *Illness as Metaphor*, pp. 21-22.
5. Ibid.; O. Carl Simonton, Stephanie Matthews-Simonton and James Creighton, *Getting Well Again*, p. 58.

over the processes involving one's body, and not knowing the causes of disease, have from time immemorial been perhaps the most disturbing aspects of illness. Belief that all diseases are actually under one's control, however unconscious the control may be, comforts the patient. Acceptance of responsibility for cancer accelerates healing through emotional tranquility, acceptance of symptoms, and avoidance of self-destructive behavior in denying the disease and not coming to terms with it.

Second, when a patient assumes responsibility for a disease, it makes the physician's job much easier, for such a patient is more peaceful and less likely to be hostile to medical authorities, who are viewed as trying to help the patient deal with his own problem. If the patient learns the concept of self-induced disease from a physician or other healer, he is likely to attribute to the healer his feeling of being in control and his improved emotional status.

The third apparent benefit of the concept is the enhanced self-esteem of patients who learn to control their feelings, or of healthy people who attribute health to their own positive attitudes. The self-potential, or human fulfillment, groups that became popular in the 1970s teach responsibility for one's own disease (or health) as a means of raising self-esteem through a sense of personal accomplishment.

But whatever the benefits of the notion of personal control over *all* health and disease, the concept is dangerous and ultimately unhealthy because it is based on an unproven premise. We simply don't know whether mental attitudes and personalities cause specific diseases, or vice versa. To ascribe diseases to a person because of personality or subconscious desires is unscientific, unfounded, and at best sheer speculation. It is the modern form of attributing disease to evil spirits. The myth discounts the possibility that things happen over which our psyches have little or no control, and makes the unwarranted assumption that our psyches can predictably and directionally influence our bodies. There is no evidence to support this supposition. Is the child who develops diabetes really at fault for the disease? It is one thing to correctly assert the nonspecific effect of emotional factors on healing, but it is quite another matter to claim that people ordain through their subconscious minds diseases which have measurable physical origins. So long as tuberculosis was essentially untreatable, its origin was explained by the myth of personality causes, but with the advent of antituberculous drugs, that particular myth has receded to deserved oblivion.

The concept of personal responsibility for health and disease is a myth because it falsely attributes natural health to ideologies, and it falsely attributes disease to individuals who usually have no control over diseases (except, of course, disease due to unhealthy habits such as drug abuse or smoking). As always, there is a price to pay for unscientific healing. Patients who have learned to believe that they unwittingly have caused their diseases are also made to feel that they deserve them.[6] The price of responsibility for one's own disease is guilt for having created it, and the burden of dealing with it. As Sontag points out, psychological theories of illness are a powerful means of placing blame on the sick,[7] and although they provide a convenient mechanism for family, friends and doctors to absolve themselves from responsibility, the process can be very unfair to the innocent patient. Also, if cure is thought to reside within the patient's mind, he is directed away from possible curative medical care or even external emotional support. By forcing patients to think of themselves as committing suicide, society solves its problem of dealing with an unwanted condition.

WHAT INDIVIDUALS CAN DO FOR THEMSELVES

There are two ways individuals can help themselves in maintaining good health: follow common-sense health rules for prevention of illness and make careful and appropriate use of health

6. Sontag, *Illness as Metaphor,* pp. 21-22.
7. Ibid.

practitioners. Fortunately, most of us are basically healthy and can maintain our health by avoiding personal and iatrogenic harm. Contrary to popular opinion, it is not necessary for us to be doing something at all times to maintain health. As Lewis Thomas has put it:

> Meanwhile, we are paying too little attention, and respect, to the built-in durability and sheer power of the human organism. Its surest tendency is toward stability and balance. It is a distortion, with something profoundly disloyal about it, to picture the human being as a teetering, fallible contraption, always needing watching and patching, always on the verge of flapping to pieces; this is the doctrine that people hear most often, and most eloquently, on all our information media.[8]

Although concepts of health maintenance through emotional attunement or natural remedies are psychologically appealing, there actually is very little beyond common-sense measures that an individual can do to maintain health. Beyond avoidance of harmful substances and habits the list thins out quickly. Except for patients with diseases which require special diets, nutrition also is a matter of common-sense avoidance of obesity and obtaining a proper mix of carbohydrate, protein and fat. There is no sound evidence that particular food supplements or vitamins can prevent anything but the rare diseases that result from specific nutritional deficiencies.

With the avalanche of claims of foods, exercises, vitamins and myriad other supposedly individual preventive measures, it is difficult to convince the public that the great source of health is communitywide preventive medicine.[9]

The many remedies which purport to promote health in already healthy people may induce a sense of personal well-feeling, but before accepting them as having actual curing effects, individuals should demand scientific evidence of benefit,

8. Lewis Thomas, *Lives of a Cell*, p. 98.
9. R.R. Rynearson, J.W. Roberts and W.L. Stewart, "Do Physician Athletes Believe in Pre-exercise Examination and Stress Tests?" *New England Journal of Medicine* 301(1979):792.

else they will be caught in the age-old trap of confusing healing with curing. Perhaps the best we can do is to live happily without an obsession about health, and investigate any new unexplained symptom by consultation with someone who has the expertise to help us.

How can individuals maximize the gains from encounters with physicians? There are many ways, but for most people it will require a substantial departure from previous methods of interacting with doctors, and a good deal of work as well. The first step is to see your doctor as you see your automobile repairman: as someone with specialized knowledge and expertise who can help you, but who possesses no magical powers. One thing is certain: If you retain the old way of thinking of a doctor as an omnipotent god, and if you continue to seek magical solutions to your problems, you will be unsuccessful in increasing your gain from visits to doctors and bettering your health.

Call your doctor "Mr.," "Mrs.," "Ms." Why do you call the physician "Dr." when you call everyone else "Mr." or "Mrs."? Why do you accord this special status? If doctors are not superhuman, wouldn't it be better to address them as you do other respected members of society?

Find out what your physician or healer can and can not do. If you go to a chiropractor, you should read extensively about chiropractors from different points of view and learn what ailments they treat best, what conditions they are unable to help, what their professional belief system is, and how they substantiate their claims. Do the same for conventional physicians. (The bibliography at the end of this book is a good place to start.) Since most people have had frequent contact with physicians and share the same medical belief system, they believe that they don't have to read about doctors to find out how they function. But when you are putting your body and your life into the hands of anyone, you serve yourself well by learning as much about his working characteristics as possible.

If you have no particular expertise in medicine, you are probably unable to judge the competence of your physician except by the outcome of your problem. In an investigation of hospital care received by Teamsters' Union members and their families, three out of four patients whose treatment was rated by reviewing specialists as substandard were convinced they had received the best possible care.[10] It is well to like your doctor and to be liked by him, but unless that is the primary purpose of the encounter, you should ascertain how successfully he accomplishes the goal of improving your health.

Understand whether you are seeking caring or curing. If curing is the goal, the claims of curing must be scrutinized, whether they come from a psychic, a chiropractor or a physician. If a holistic healer is appealing because you feel the need for harmony between mind and body and a return to more honest and natural values, you must ask whether this is sufficient or whether physical curing is necessary as well. You must ask yourself whether your choice of a healer is determined by attraction to a compatible life-philosophy, or whether a less pleasant physical approach to biological dysfunction is in order.

Learn not to substitute curing for caring. Find out what your problem is, and whether it requires curative therapy or whether you can heal yourself with sufficient emotional support. *Never, never* insist upon or ask for or even suggest curative therapy if your doctor has not already done so. If a physician finds nothing wrong, but you want to feel better, go to a masseuse or talk to a friend, but don't shop for an operation. Learn not to couch psychological problems in somatic terms. If you are upset over a family matter and have a headache as well, tell the doctor about your emotional state as well as your headache. If you want warmth and consideration and caring, fine—go get it; but don't confuse it with curative medical care. Keep as your goal avoidance of curative therapies unless they are absolutely necessary.

10. Spencer Klaw, *The Great American Medicine Show*, p. 98.

When a cure is necessary, be sure that the one you get has been well tested —ask for the facts. In considering a major therapy that is potentially fatal or injurious, try to eliminate emotional considerations; a dangerous procedure shouldn't be applied without caring, but the desire for caring or healing should not interfere with proper application of curative therapy. Make your doctor know that you respect his opinion, but that you want the facts as well, and that you can tell the difference. Keep in mind that you can never fully inform yourself about your medical problem unless you go through medical school first, and even then, like many doctors, you would not know everything about most illnesses and treatments.

Insist on being an equal partner in all decisions, using the doctor's knowledge and skills but not giving him control over you. Remember always that the best-intentioned doctor can have financial and professional interests that are in conflict with your own, and if you and your physician do not minimize these conflicts, you will be the worse for it. You want your medical care to be patient-centered, not doctor-centered.

Do not follow the recommendations of a physician who stands to profit from his decisions until you have checked them out with an independent consultant who does not have the same interests and incentives as the first doctor. The person who gets the very best medical care is the one who has a family member or close friend who is a physician and will oversee all decisions. You need a similar physician advocate. If you don't have one in your family or among your friends, your best bet is the family practice physician, one who knows you well enough to take the information supplied by a specialist and use it in conjunction with your medical history to suggest the best course of action.

Society ought to insist that the profession develop patient-advocate physicians, primary physicians whose economic and professional incentives would be patient-oriented. Each patient should have such a physician who would be responsible for all medical treatment, except for emergencies when he is not available or not expert enough to counsel the patient. This new breed of physician[11] would have the authority within the profession to make, with the patient, all medical decisions, including those requiring the use of advanced technology and specialized surgical procedures. He would use the expert advice of specialists, who would appropriately be seen as technicians able to diagnose disease in their special fields and perform necessary procedures. The primary physician would be expert in acquiring and interpreting data so as to be able to make well-informed decisions in all areas of medicine. With the resources of modern medicine to draw on but free from the myth of the healer, he could perform the three most humanitarian functions of a doctor: to comfort, to teach and to provide curative therapy when necessary.

11. B.F. Fuller and Frank Fuller, *Physician or Magician?*, p. 18.

Bibliography

BOOKS

Annas, George J. *The Rights of Hospital Patients: An American Civil Liberties Union Handbook.* New York: Avon Books, 1975.

Berman, Edgar. *The Solid Gold Stethoscope.* New York: Ballantine Books, 1976.

Bloom, Samuel. *The Doctor and His Patient.* New York: The Free Press, 1965.

Blum, Richard H.; Sadusk, J.; and Waterson, R. *The Management of the Doctor-Patient Relationship.* New York: McGraw-Hill Book Co., 1960.

Boas, Franz. *The Religion of the Kwakiutl Indians.* Part 2, *Translations.* New York: Columbia University Press, 1930.

Bok, Sissela. *Lying: Moral Choice in Public and Private Life.* New York: Vintage Books, 1978.

Bosk, Charles. *Forgive and Remember: Managing Medical Failure.* Chicago: University of Chicago Press, 1979.

Bronowski, J. *The Common Sense of Science.* Cambridge: Harvard University Press, 1978.

Bunker, John P., et al., eds. *Costs, Risks, and Benefits of Surgery.* New York: Oxford University Press, 1977.

Camp, John. *The Healer's Art: The Doctor Through History.* New York: Taplinger Publishing Co., 1977.

Carlson, Rick J. *The End of Medicine.* New York: John Wiley & Sons, Inc., 1975.

Cassell, Eric. *The Healer's Art.* Philadelphia: J.B. Lippincott Company, 1976.

Cousins, Norman. *Anatomy of an Illness.* New York: W.W. Norton Co., Inc., 1979.

Crile, George. *Surgery: Your Choices, Your Alternatives.* New York: Delacorte Press/Seymour Lawrence, 1978.

Dixon, Bernard. *Beyond the Magic Bullet.* New York: Harper & Row, 1978.

Dollery, Colin. *The End of an Age of Optimism.* London: The Nuffield Provincial Hospitals Trust, 1978.

Dubos, René. *Man Adapting.* New Haven: Yale University Press, 1965.

Ellison, David. *The Bio-Medical Fix.* Westport, Conn.: Greenwood Press, 1978.

Engelhardt, H. Tristram; Spicker, Stuart; and Towers, Bernard. *Clinical Judgment: A Critical Appraisal.* Boston: D. Reidel Publishing Company, 1979.

Fox, Renee C., and Swazey, Judith P. *The Courage to Fail.* Chicago: University of Chicago Press, 1974.

Frank, Jerome D. *Persuasion and Healing.* New York: Schocken Books, 1974.

Freidson, Eliot. *Profession of Medicine.* New York: Dodd, Mead & Co., 1975.

Fuchs, Victor R. *Who Shall Live?* New York: Basic Books, 1974.

Fuller, B.F., and Fuller, Frank. *Physician or Magician?* Washington, D.C.: Hemisphere Publishing Corporation, 1978.

Gallagher, Eugene, ed. *The Doctor-Patient Relationship in the Changing Health Scene.* DHEW Publication No. (NIH) 78-183. Washington, D.C.: Government Printing Office, 1978.

Ginzberg, Eli. *The Limits of Health Reform.* New York: Basic Books, 1977.

Grossinger, Richard. *Planet Medicine.* Garden City, N.Y.: Anchor Press/Doubleday, 1980.

Hamilton, Edith. *Mythology: Timeless Tales of Gods and Heroes.* New York: Mentor Books, 1961.

Hill, Austin B. *Statistical Methods in Clinical and Preventive Medicine.* Edinburgh: Livingstone, 1962.

[Hippocrates]. *The Genuine Works of Hippocrates.* Trans. Francis Adams. New York: William Wood and Company, 1886. Two vols.

Holmes, Oliver Wendell. *Currents and Counter-Currents in Medical Science.* Boston: Ticknor & Fields, 1861.

———. *Medical Essays: 1842-1882.* 1893. Reprint. Darby, Pa.: Arden Library, 1977.

Illich, Ivan. *Medical Nemesis: The Expropriation of Health.* New York: Bantam Books, Inc., 1976.

Jonas, Steven. *Medical Mystery.* New York: W.W. Norton Co., Inc., 1978.

Jonsen, Albert R. *The Rights of Physicians: A Philosophical Essay.* Washington, D.C.: Institute of Medicine, 1978.

Klaw, Spencer. *The Great American Medicine Show.* New York: Penguin Books, 1976.

Knowles, John H., ed. *Doing Better and Feeling Worse.* New York: W.W. Norton Co., Inc., 1977.

Kuhn, Thomas. *The Structure of Scientific Revolutions.* 2nd ed. Chicago: University of Chicago Press, 1970.

Lear, Martha, *Heart Sounds.* New York: Simon and Schuster, 1980.

Lewis, Sinclair. *Arrowsmith*. New York: New American Library, 1961.

Lipp, Martin. *The Bitter Pill*. New York, Harper & Row, 1980.

McKeown, Thomas. *The Role of Medicine: Dream, Mirage, or Nemesis?* Princeton: Princeton University Press, 1979.

Mason, Steven F. *A History of the Sciences*. New York: Collier Books, 1962.

Mechanic, David. *Future Issues in Health Care*. New York: The Free Press, 1979.

Meek, George W. *Healers and the Healing Process*. Wheaton, Ill.: The Theosophical Publishing House, 1977.

Mendelsohn, Robert S. *Confessions of a Medical Heretic*. Chicago: Contemporary Books, 1979.

Millman, Marcia. *The Unkindest Cut*. New York: William Morrow and Co., 1977.

Mills, George S. *Rogues and Heroes from Iowa's Amazing Past*. Ames: Iowa State University Press, 1972.

Mullin, Fitzhugh. *White Coat, Clenched Fist*. New York: Macmillan, 1976.

Murphy, Edmond A. *The Logic of Medicine*. Baltimore: Johns Hopkins University Press, 1976.

Nolen, William A. *Healing: A Doctor in Search of a Miracle*. Greenwich: Fawcett Publications, Inc., 1974.

Parsons, Talcott. *The Social System*. Glencoe, Ill.: The Free Press, 1951.

Pearson, Karl. *The Grammar of Science*. 2nd ed. London: Adam and Charles Black, 1900.

Popper, Karl. *The Logic of Scientific Discovery*. New York: Harper & Row, 1968.

Preston, Thomas A. *Coronary Artery Surgery: A Critical Review*. New York: Raven Press, 1977.

Reiser, S.J. *Medicine and the Reign of Technology*. Cambridge: Cambridge University Press, 1978.

Rushmer, Robert. *Humanizing Health Care: Alternative Futures for Medicine*. Cambridge, Mass.: The MIT Press, 1978.

Shaw, George Bernard. *The Doctor's Dilemma*. Baltimore: Penguin Books, 1954.

Shem, Samuel. *The House of God*. New York: Richard Marek Publishers, 1978.

Shryock, Richard H. *Medicine in America*. Baltimore: Johns Hopkins Press, 1966.

Sigerist, Henry E. *The Great Doctors*. 2nd ed. New York: W.W. Norton Co., Inc. 1933.

_____. *Medicine and Human Welfare.* New Haven: Yale University Press, 1941.

Simonton, O. Carl; Matthews-Simonton, Stephanie; and Creighton, James. *Getting Well Again.* Los Angeles: J.P. Tarcher, 1978.

Singer, Charles, and Underwood, Ashworth E. *A Short History of Medicine.* 2nd ed. New York: Oxford University Press, 1962.

Sontag, Susan. *Illness as Metaphor.* New York: Vintage Books, 1979.

Strauss, Anselm, and Howard, Jan. *Humanizing Health Care.* New York: John Wiley & Sons, 1975.

Swazey, Judith P. *Health, Professionals, and the Public: Toward a New Social Contract?* Philadelphia: Society of Health and Human Values, 1979.

Thomas, Lewis. *The Lives of a Cell.* New York: Bantam Books, Inc., 1975.

_____. *The Medusa and the Snail.* New York: Viking Press, 1979.

Whitehead, Alfred North. *Science and the Modern World.* New York: Mentor Books, 1948.

Williams, Robert. *To Live and To die: When, Why, and How.* New York: Springer-Verlag, 1973.

Young, James H. *The Medical Messiahs.* Princeton: Princeton University Press, 1967.

ARTICLES

Almy, Thomas P. "The Role of the Primary Physician in the Health-Care 'Industry.'" *New England Journal of Medicine* 304(1981):225-28.

Beaty, H.N. and Petersdorf, R.G. "Iatrogenic Factors in Infectious Disease." *Annals of Internal Medicine* 65(1966):641-55.

Berg, A.O., and LoGerfo, J.P. "Potential Effect of Self-Care Algorithms on the Number of Physician Visits." *New England Journal of Medicine* 300(1979):535-37.

Bergman, A.B., and Stamm, S.J. "The Morbidity of Cardiac Non-Disease in Schoolchildren." *New England Journal of Medicine* 276(1967): 1008-13.

Bibbo, M. "Follow-Up Study of Male and Female Offspring of DES-Exposed Mothers." *Journal of Obstetrics and Gynecology* 49(1977):1-8.

Blendon, R.J. "Can China's Health Care Be Transplanted Without China's Economic Policies?" *New England Journal of Medicine* 300(1979):1453-58.

"Breast-Cancer Management." *New England Journal of Medicine* 301(1979):326-28.

Bunker, J.P. "Surgical Manpower: A Comparison of Operations and Surgeons in the United States and in England and Wales." *New England Journal of Medicine* 282(1970):135-44.

Bunker, J.P. "When the Medical Interests of Society Are in Conflict with Those of the Individual, Who Wins?" *Pharos* 39(1976):64-66.

Bunker, J.P., and Brown, B.W. "The Physician-Patient as an Informed Consumer of Surgical Services." *New England Journal of Medicine* 290(1974):1051-55.

Burch, G.E. "Of 'Now Myocardial Imaging.'" *American Heart Journal* 99(1980):540.

Cay, E.L., et al. "Patient's Assessment of the Result of Surgery for Peptic Ulcer." *Lancet* 1(1975):29-31.

Chapman, C.B. "On the Definition and Teaching of the Medical Ethic." *New England Journal of Medicine* 301(1979):630-38.

"Chiropractic: Recognized but Unproven." *New England Journal of Medicine* 301(1979):659-60.

Crile, George. "The Surgeon's Dilemma." *Harper's Magazine* 250 (1975):30-38.

Delbanco, T.L.; Meyers, K.C.; and Segal, E.A. "Paying the Physician's Fee." *New England Journal of Medicine* 301(1979):1314-20.

"Doctors' Fees—Free from the Law of Supply and Demand." *Science* 200(1978):30.

Dunea, G. "Healing by Touching." *British Medical Journal* 1 (1979):795-96.

Dunn, P.M. "Obstetric Delivery Today: For Better or for Worse?" *Lancet* 1(1976):790-93.

Enthoven, A.C. "Cutting Cost Without Cutting the Quality of Care." *New England Journal of Medicine* 298(1978):1229-38.

"An Ethical Consideration of Large-Scale Clinical Trials in Cardiovascular Diseases." Report of the Committee on Ethics of the American Heart Association. *Circulation* 52(1975):pages 5-9.

Fish, R.G.; Crymes, T.P.; and Lovell, M.G. "Internal Mammary Artery Ligation for Angina Pectoris." *New England Journal of Medicine* 259(1958):418-20.

Frankfurter, Felix. "A Lawyer's Dicta on Doctors." *Harvard Medical Alumni Bulletin,* (July 1958), pp. 12-17.

Glantz, S.A. "Biostatistics: How to Detect, Correct and Prevent Errors in the Medical Literature." *Circulation* 61(1980):1-7.

Gliedman, L.H.; Gantt, W.H.; and Teitelbaum, H.A. "Some Implications of Conditional Reflex Studies for Placebo Research." *American Journal of Psychiatry* 113(1957):1102-1107.

Harrison, T.R. "The Value and Limitation of Laboratory Tests in Clinical Medicine." *Journal of the Medical Association of Alabama* 13(1944):381-84.

Holden, C. "FDA Tells Senators of Doctors Who Fake Data in Clinical Trials." *Science* 206(1979):432-33.

Holman, H.R. "The 'Excellence' Deception in Medicine." *Hospital Practice* 11(1976):11-21.

"How Much Government Control Do We Really Need?" *Drug Therapy* 8(1978):7.

Ingelfinger, F.J. "Health: A Matter of Statistics or Feeling?" *New England Journal of Medicine* 296(1977):448-49.

———. "Medicine: Meritorious or Meretricious." *Science* 200(1978): 942-46.

Levine, J.D.; Gordon, N.C.; and Fields, H.L. "The Mechanism of Placebo Anesthesia." *Lancet* 2(1978):654-57.

Luce, J.M. "Chiropractic—Its History and Challenge to Medicine." *Pharos* 41(1978):12-17.

McCarthy, E.G. "Effects of Screening by Consultants on Recommended Elective Surgical Procedures." *New England Journal of Medicine* 291(1974):133-35.

McQueen, D.V. "The History of Science and Medicine as Theoretical Sources of the Comparative Study of Contemporary Medical Systems." *Social Science and Medicine* 12(2B)(1978):69-77.

Mahler, H. "Health—A Demystification of Medical Technology." *Lancet* 2(1975):829-33.

Mantle, J.A., et al. "Emergency Revascularization for Acute Myocardial Infarction: An Unproved Experimental Approach." *American Journal of Cardiology* 44(1979):1407-1409.

Moss, J.E. "Congressional Scrutiny Reveals Sore Spots of U.S. Health Care." *Legal Aspects of Medical Practice* 6(1978):28-31.

N.I.H. Conference. "Basic and Clinical Studies of Endorphins." *Annals of Internal Medicine* 91(1979):229-50.

Relman, A.S. "The Allocation of Medical Resources by Physicians." *Journal of Medical Education* 55(1980):99-104.

Rich, Howard H. "How Much Government Control Do We Really Need?" *Drug Therapy* 8(1978):7.

Rifkin, S.B. "Politics of Barefoot Medicine." *Lancet* 1(1978):34.

Robin, E.D. "Overdiagnosis and Overtreatment of Pulmonary Embolism: The Emperor May Have No Clothes." *Annals of Internal Medicine* 87(1977):775-81.

Rosenweig, A.L. "Iatrogenic Anemia." *Archives of Internal Medicine* 138(1978):1843.

Rynearson, R.R.; Roberts, J.W.; and Stewart, W.L. "Do Physician Athletes Believe in Pre-exercise Examination and Stress Tests?" *New England Journal of Medicine* 301(1979):792-93.

Schor, S., and Karten, L. "Statistical Evaluation of Medical Manuscripts." *Journal of the American Medical Association* 195 (1966):1123-28.

Schroeder, S.A.; Marton, K.I.; and Strom, B.L. "Frequency and Morbidity of Invasive Procedures." *Archives of Internal Medicine* 138(1978):1809-11.

Sheehan, T.J. "The Medical Literature: Let the Reader Beware." *Archives of Internal Medicine* 140(1980):472-74.

Siegler, M., and Osmond, H. "Aesculapian Authority." *Hastings Center Studies* 1(1973):41-52.

Sloan, F., and Steinwald, B. "Determinants of Physicians' Fees." *Journal of Business* 47(1974):493-511.

Soffer, A. "Consumer's Rights in Medicine." *Archives of Internal Medicine* 138(1978):905.

Sosa, R., et al. "The Effect of a Supportive Companion on Perinatal Problems, Length of Labor, and Mother-Infant Interaction." *New England Journal of Medicine* 303(1980):597-600.

Steele, K., et al. "Iatrogenic Illness on a General Medical Service at a University Hospital." *New England Journal of Medicine* 304 (1981):638-42.

Szasz, Thomas S., and Hollender, M.H. "The Basic Models of the Doctor-Patient Relationship." *Archives of Internal Medicine* 97 (1956):585-92.

Vayda, E. "A Comparison of Surgical Rates in Canada and in England and Wales." *New England Journal of Medicine* 289(1973):1224-29.

Wennberg, J., and Gittlesohn, A. "Small Area Variations in Health Care Delivery." *Science* 182(1973):1102-1108.

Index